THE 3-WEEK FAMILY FAT CURE

EMMAUS PUBLIC LIBRARY
11 EAST MAIN STREET
EMMAUS, PA 18049

THE 3-WEEK FAMILY FAT CURE

You Don't Have to Be Overweight
Just Because Your Parents Are

JOHN MAYER, Ph.D

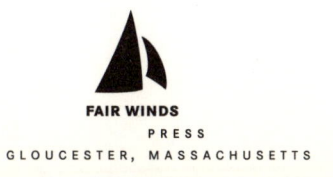

FAIR WINDS
PRESS
GLOUCESTER, MASSACHUSETTS

Text © John E. Mayer, Ph.D.

First published in the USA in 2003 by
Fair Winds Press
33 Commercial Street
Gloucester, MA 01930

All rights reserved. No part of this book may be reproduced or utilized, in any form or by any means, electronic or mechanical, without prior permission in writing from the publisher.

Cover design by Laura Shaw Design
Book design by *tabula rasa* graphic design

Printed and bound in Canada

Library of Congress Cataloging-in-Publication Data

Mayer, John E., [date]
    The 3-week family fat cure : the revolutionary family fit program that breaks the cycle of obesity for good / John E. Mayer.
        p.;   cm.
    Includes bibliographical references.
    ISBN 1-931412-02-2
    1. Family—Health and hygiene. 2. Overweight persons—Family relationships. 3. Obesity—Prevention. 4. Physical fitness. 5. Diet. 6. Health.
[DNLM: 1. Obesity—prevention & control—Popular Works. 2. Behavior Therapy—methods—Popular Works. 3. Eating—Popular Works. 4. Family Therapy—methods—Popular Works. WD 212 M4675z 2002] I. Title: Three-week family fat cure. II. Title: Revolutionary family fit program that breaks the cycle of obesity for good. III. Title.
RA777.7 .M39 2002
616.3'9805—dc21   2002008169

10 9 8 7 6 5 4 3 2 1

The information in this book is for educational purposes only. It is not intended to replace the advice of a physician or medical practitioner. Please see your health care provider before beginning any new health program.

ACKNOWLEDGMENTS

First, thanks to my family for putting up with even less of me while working on this book. To my fitness colleague, John O'Connor, for being supportive and open to bouncing ideas back and forth. To the whole O'Connor clan, Kelly, Jennifer, Catherine, Megan, and Danny, for being a Family Fit family.

To Barbara Neighbors Deal, who saw the value of this book immediately and convinced others to believe in it also.

To Holly Schmidt, who knew what she wanted from the beginning. To Wendy Simard, who shepherded the project along until excellence unfolded.

Finally, to all of the families I have encountered in my professional work. They have always taught me what they needed, and I had the wisdom to listen and help.

To my family: my wife Deborah, and children Courtney and Justin. You are the inspiration, models, and motivation for developing this program and putting it into a book. You are the best examples of Family Fit, the best people I know, and my best friends.

CONTENTS

Introduction	Escaping the "Fat" Label	1
PART I	**Generations of Obesity**	
Chapter 1	Families and the Painful Cycle of Obesity	11
Chapter 2	Why Are We All Fat?	23
PART II	**The Big Picture**	
Chapter 3	Preparing for the Program	39
Chapter 4	The Program Overview: The Three Pillars	61
PART III	**Three Weeks and Three Ways to Success: The Family Fit Program**	
Chapter 5	The First Way—The Diet and Nutrition Pillar	95
Chapter 6	The Second Way—Motivating Generations to Change	130
Chapter 7	The Third Way—Family Fitness Activity	143
PART IV	**Staying on the Program**	
Chapter 8	Triggers That Lead Back to Bad Habits	165
Chapter 9	A Short Course on Parenting	173
Chapter 10	Positive Side Effects	187
PART V	**Real Generations**	
Chapter 11	Success Stories	197
Chapter 12	Family Fitness Myths and Facts	211
Chapter 13	Outside Resources for the Family	219
Bibliography		223
About the Author		237

INTRODUCTION

Escaping the "Fat" Label

I was a fat child. My mom was fat, my dad was fat, and my grandparents were fat. Every picture in our house documented generations of obese relatives. These images surrounded me as I grew up. I was handed a legacy of entrapment into a world of struggle with weight.

As a child born into this legacy, I did fat things. I ate fat foods. I shopped at fat stores. I did fat activities. Most painful of all, I was the brunt of every cruel fat insult imaginable. Some of these insults were intentional, as when attacked by peers. Other insults were unintentional, as when assaulted by well-meaning adults. The common adult remark I heard was, "Oh, my, what a big boy! He's so nice looking and he'll lose all that baby fat." These adult remarks were just as painful as those of my playmates, such as "Hey, Lardo!" or "Fatty-fatty two-by-four, can't get through the kitchen door." I was not a happy child.

I did not do well in school. The fat boy is expected to be the class clown, and I filled that role expertly by getting into trouble frequently in the primary grades. My pranks culminated in having my diploma handed to my parents outside of the graduation ceremony.

Like most fat kids, when I wanted to break away from my family destiny, the response from my family was based on wisdom handed down to them from previous generations. If my family discovered that I was dieting, they made me feel guilty and embarrassed. This was not my family's fault; the concept of a ten-year-old feeling hurt by his weight simply was not in the parenting handbook their parents gave them. Most often my family's comments on losing weight were, "Don't be silly, eat, you're just big boned" or "You've got a lot of baby fat; that goes away. Now stop being stupid and eat." At this early age I felt a hopelessness that life had thrown me a handicap I could never overcome.

My parents were warm, loving people who took their greatest joys in life from seeing their children happy. But even with this strong bond they couldn't understand or help with the suffering I was living with. As a result, I learned early on not to share this pain with them. The script they received as parents told them that children must be fed well so that they will thrive and be strong. A big appetite in a child was a badge of good parenting. It was understandable that my parents couldn't empathize with the pain I was going through as a fat child trapped inside a body and an image I didn't want.

When I did make my escape from the prison of obesity, I did it in a dangerous way. It was the summer before entering high school, and I was determined not to start high school as a "fat boy" and endure even worse taunts and embarrassment in the powerful teenage social pecking order. I did not want to repeat the experiences I had in elementary school. Even though others viewed me as a jovial, popular playmate, I was sad and lonely inside. I knew something made me different, and the obvious sign of that difference was my fat body. That summer the idea of my "great escape" from obesity came to my naïve mind. My plan was to simply not eat while addicting myself to a daily routine of playing sports with friends. I would keep my escape hidden from my parents by staying out all day. They would never know if I ate.

My fat poured off. When I started my great escape, the next pair of jeans I was going to buy would have been a size 40 waist. By the time I entered high school I was wearing a size 29 waist, and I was proudly carrying the athlete's V shape of broad shoulders tapering to a thin waist. My great escape was successful, but luckily I was physically strong. I could have seriously hurt myself in the process from the punishment I was putting my body through.

My new body led to a new cycle of personal success. Looking like an athlete dictated that I become an athlete in high school. By changing my body, I developed strong self-confidence from accomplishing what I had thought was an impossible feat. This self-confidence perpetuated further accomplishments and built solid self-esteem. My high school years were successful and happy. I did well in school and changed my image from one of a class clown to one of a leader/scholar/athlete. Those years built a foundation that culminated in overcoming other obstacles, gaining entrance into medical school, and launching a successful professional career.

Sadly, my parents never fully embraced my new lifestyle. Because I was forced to accomplish my great escape alone, they never knew the magnitude of the accomplishment and how it became the cornerstone of other successes. They were proud of me and my accomplishments with my body, but they did not single out my fitness lifestyle for special recognition. In their minds, they believed the old wisdom that baby fat disappears in due time. They had no idea what commitment and hardship it took for the fat to disappear.

My example of weight control and fitness never rubbed off on them when I was young. Many years later each of my parents had their own epiphanies that led them to healthier lifestyles. For each of them this was because of a serious health scare. They tried in their own ways to eat healthier and to become more physically active, but they could never shake the generations of messages that threw them back into bad habits.

My father tried to eat better foods, but he couldn't break the habit of eating large quantities of food. He continued to be obese. To this day in my own family we call overeating "Grandpa Mayer Disease."

My mother was by nature a very tiny woman. She was well under five feet tall, and she had feet so small that she could buy her shoes in the children's department of stores. As an adult she wore a size 16 dress for as far back as I can remember. After her resolution to eat healthier and become more active, she didn't have to fight Grandpa Mayer Disease; instead, she kept her weight up by never altering her love affair with high-calorie, fattening sweets and desserts. She believed that these "treats" were her reward for exercising and eating better main courses.

The discovery of the successful program described in this book obviously did not come from my parents; instead, it arose out of my own professional life and parenting my own family with a wonderful, special spouse who loves life and family.

As fate would have it, my career led me to a specialty in helping people with addictions. One of my first professional positions involved designing and implementing a program to help severely overweight people rapidly lose weight before mandatory surgery. My own struggle with obesity was instrumental in understanding the needs of overweight individuals and the prison they live in because of the generations of behaviors that they have inherited.

This book fills the need to give families a straightforward solution to the generational cycle of obesity. The popular diet programs that appear in print do not address obesity across the life span. A review of the best-selling diet books published over the last decade showed that only three even mentioned the critical developmental years when obesity takes root. No mention is made in any of these books of the problem of obesity across generations or the contribution that generational family patterns make to the cycle of obesity.

The highly successful program described in this book begins with accepting the fact that obesity is an often crippling disorder that has its roots in childhood and has many causes. Breaking out of the grip of obesity must involve a multifaceted approach that surrounds the individual with new lifestyle choices. For a weight loss program to be successful, it must recognize that eating and food are pleasurable human activities. To try to convince a person that eating is not pleasurable is unrealistic. Weight loss programs based on denying one the pleasure of food and stressing sacrifice are *negatively centered programs.*

This book centers on accepting a positive attitude toward eating. The program is enjoyable and doable for every family member. It recognizes that food is one of life's primary pleasures. Eating is physically, emotionally, and socially pleasing in ways that no other activity can match.

From a sociological perspective, eating and dining have traditionally been basic ways that families socialize and communicate. No other human activity is as emotionally charged as the act of eating. Psychologists know that eating is one of the two primary human reinforcements, and because of survival needs it ranks higher than the other reinforcement (sex). Programs that try to change people's eating habits must first accept the primary importance and pleasure of eating in each human and collectively in families.

Similarly, to be successful we must accept the fact that many forces push family members to be overweight. These forces are heredity, society, instinct, emotions, and family habits. To deny the existence of either the pleasure of eating or these many forces is a sure road to failure. Denying both of these facts is a handicap that no weight loss program can overcome.

Historically, diet programs have not recognized the powerful importance of eating. These programs have thought of eating as a negative habit or a nuisance. The techniques offered by these programs have predictably followed that thinking and have stressed sacrifice and denial. By emphasizing this negatively centered approach, these programs cannot be successful over time. Because of this long-term failure, the dieter is then left no choice but to try the next fad diet from an ever-expanding market of programs. The revolving door of obesity just keeps moving round and round.

The current scientific research on obesity supports the view that these negatively centered approaches to dieting contribute to the roller coaster of weight loss and weight gain. The program here is centered on a positive recognition of the importance of food and eating as a primary part of the human condition. This program is not afraid to apply the word "fun" to dieting. This program alters negative eating behaviors and changes the social/emotional forces that contribute to obesity in each family member regardless of age. Furthermore, because of the foundation of positive, enjoyable change, families of any makeup can successfully use this program. Single-parent families, blended families, and traditional families can use the program because it is easy and fits into the time demands of the modern family. The program detailed in this book is directed at the health needs of people across the life span. This makes this book useful to all people—from great-grandparents to great-grandchildren.

PART I
GENERATIONS OF OBESITY

CHAPTER ONE

Families and the Painful Cycle of Obesity

Jack was thirteen and living in a midwestern city. He was a handsome boy with classic features and a clear, ruddy complexion. Jack was tall for his age—five foot eight and a half in the seventh grade. Jack was also considerably overweight. He wasn't "Fat Albert" fat, but his clothes couldn't hide the fact that he had rolls of fat around his waistline and that his chest was shaped more like a woman's breasts than like the flat, strong plates of the male athlete he dreamt of becoming.

The femalelike chest bothered Jack the most. Those flabby protrusions on his chest saddened him. He thought about his fleshy chest every day. To try to cover up his condition, Jack wore undershirts one size too small because he thought that this flattened his chest.

The undershirt trick wasn't the only maneuver that Jack used to cover up his fat. He also had chubby cheeks. That year, in the seventh grade, he started a new habit of slightly sucking in his cheeks constantly to give his face a thinner, more angular shape. He tried holding in his stomach, too, but his underdeveloped abdominal muscles couldn't maintain the contraction for any length of time so he quickly gave this up.

At school, boys and girls were already pairing off into "couples." They used the term "going out," but most of their parents didn't allow them to date at such an early age, so they didn't actually go out together. Jack was not chosen to "go out" with any of the girls, and he was too self-conscious of his body shape to ask a girl to do so. Jack faced this painful reality every day at school because he sat next to Sharon, the girl he, and most of the other boys, most wanted to "go out" with.

Sharon was one of those wholesomely pretty girls who didn't have to do anything to make herself one of the most attractive girls in the seventh grade. Her personality matched her effortless looks. She was very open and friendly to everyone, especially to her desk partner, Jack. Instead of pleasing Jack, her friendliness actually made Jack feel worse about himself because he believed Sharon might go out with him if only he weren't so overweight. Still, Jack hoped that things could be different.

One day was particularly torturous for Jack. Sharon began to discreetly lift her uniform skirt in class and whispered to Jack, "I want to show you something special." Jack's heart pounded, and he allowed himself once more to entertain the possibility that he could be part of a couple just like other boys his age. When her skirt reached mid-thigh, her leg revealed a set of initials drawn with a ballpoint pen. Shock ran through Jack's heart like a full-blown heart attack, for the initials weren't his. The initials were those of another classmate, who wasn't a handsome lad. Even Jack, blanketed with the ingrained humility from his upbringing, felt he was better looking than this other boy. Jack was left with only one conclusion—the only attraction Sharon could have for this other boy was his body shape. He was thin and athletic, and Jack wasn't. Jack, a tough, urban adolescent, went home that day and cried for the first time since he was five years old.

Looking back at Jack's pain with the eyes and mind of an adult, we could suggest all kinds of remedies for the pain that Jack suffered daily as a result of his weight. But Jack was a thirteen-year-old boy who lived with his parents. Both of Jack's parents had Jack's body shape. They were tall for their generation and they were considerably obese. Like Jack, his parents weren't grossly obese, but each was at least thirty pounds overweight.

Jack's genes set the table for his lifelong struggles with weight. Jack couldn't prepare his own meals or choose the foods he ate. That was unheard of in his family at any age, let alone at thirteen. His parents' attitude was, what does a thirteen-year-old know about what he should eat? So Jack ate the rich, ethnic foods that had been handed down for generations in his family. Almost all of these foods did not help Jack's weight problem one bit.

Even when a young person like Jack is aware of a solution to his problems, he may be helpless to change his fate when surrounded by forces that lock him into an unhealthy lifestyle. In Jack's situation, in spite of an environment that imprisoned him in his fat body, Jack tried to control his weight. In Jack's young but perceptive mind, that meant only one avenue—lessening the total amount of food he ate. He didn't know about calories or nutritional counts, but it made sense to him that the less you eat, the less you gain. Even though Jack was a very bright and socially aware child, the concept of toning his body by physical activity never entered his mind. How could it? Jack's parents did not exercise; in fact, they led very sedentary lives. The family's favorite forms of recreation were, in order: watching television, talking on the telephone, dining out at fast-food restaurants, and watching a movie on occasion. Jack was not introduced to exercise until junior high school gym class, and that experience was a sham. The teacher "taught" the class by throwing a ball down on the gym floor and barking at the students to play for fifty minutes. The ball would change with each season, but the routine stayed the same. Exercise and physical activity were not taught as a lifestyle but were presented as just another form of chaotic school recess.

So Jack was left with attempting to look like the boy he dreamed of becoming by eating less food. But even here his environment stymied Jack. Several times while he was in the sixth grade (he was about eleven or twelve years old), Jack sat at the dinner table and did not eat all the food that was heaped on his plate. When this occurred he received a stern reprimand from both of his parents as well as cruel taunting from his siblings. His parents would say, "You're going to get sick if you don't eat all of your food. Now eat everything on that plate or you cannot leave the table." And "Don't be wasteful. Mother worked hard to prepare that food, and Dad works hard to allow us to pay for that food. How can you be so bad as to not finish your plate?"

Jack's siblings jumped at the opportunity to goad Jack by saying, "Oh, Jackie, trying to kiss a girl. So you found out they don't kiss fat boys." And "Ohhh…little fat Jackie is on a girlie diet…trying to be Miss America?"

The pain from his weight wasn't confined to being hurt in his relationships with girls. Somehow, half of Jack's four brothers and sisters had managed to avoid the obesity that plagues this family. Those siblings of average weight teased Jack constantly, chiding him with sarcasm and names that replaced common communication or were effortlessly added to everyday conversation. Even Jack's best friend didn't call him by name, but always greeted Jack with slang meant to be friendly or funny but which hurt Jack to his core. Jack's buddy most commonly greeted him with "Hi, Fat" or "Hey, Big Boy." Jack never told his friend how much those words hurt. After all, Jack thought to do so would leave him without a friend, and then he would be all alone—no girlfriend and no male pals to hang with either. So Jack went along with all the fat taunts and even participated in them at times just to be accepted, and the cycle of obesity continued for him.

The Obesity Epidemic

Jack's pain opens a window onto a condition that thousands of young people suffer with each day in the United States. We saw just a few small glimpses of the pain that surrounds Jack everywhere he turns in his young life. In the past if we have thought about weight, eating, and the desire to be thinner among young people, we were made aware of the hardships of girls. We were lulled into thinking that if weight problems existed in our youth, they must be the problem of young girls: They are seduced by the bold images created by the media, but these females will outgrow this foolishness somehow. We now know how wrong this thinking actually is. Obesity is an epidemic in children of both sexes and in whole families. It is an epidemic that is growing out of control. Males are just as seduced by the dream to be thinner as females. They are surrounded by images that idealize the American athlete or the emaciated rock 'n' roll star. Even though statistics have shown for years that males are just as affected by obesity as females, we haven't often considered the feelings of boys like Jack as they grow up in a world that presses them to be athletic looking and lean even as it screams at them to overeat and overlounge.

The Surgeon General's office estimates that 14 percent of our children are overweight. That figure is *triple* what it was in the sixties. Furthermore, of those children that are overweight, they are 20 percent to 30 percent heavier than they were ten years ago. The number of overweight black and Hispanic children has doubled over the last ten years to just over 22 percent of all children in these ethnic groups. At the same time, the number of overweight Caucasian children in this same ten-year period has risen by 50 percent to include 12 percent of all Caucasian children.

To highlight the significance of these figures, the estimated number of youths with drug problems is approximately 10 percent. This makes obesity in children a larger social problem than drugs in our youth by approximately 50 percent. Society is shocked to discover drug problems in youth, yet the larger problem of obesity barely gets a raised eyebrow in some communities.

Our children did not get this way in a vacuum. The Surgeon General's recent report on obesity revealed that *60 percent* of adults are overweight or obese! In addition, three hundred thousand Americans die each year from illnesses caused or worsened by obesity. This number of deaths attributable to a preventable cause will soon overtake tobacco as the chief cause of death. If one in seven children are overweight—and this is what these statistics amount to—then they are surrounded by about five in seven adults who are overweight. Seeing such a large percentage of overweight adults surrounding them, overweight children are more likely to resign themselves to their body condition as simply the way of the world. There can be no doubt that obesity is a painful cycle that becomes a family's self-fulfilling prophecy generation after generation.

Adults establish households with lifestyles and philosophies based on how they live in this world. If 60 percent of American adults are overweight, that means that the majority of households in this country are being led into a cycle of poor eating and lack of exercise that will increase these numbers in the future. Think about it. Probability theory tells us that outcomes can be mathematically determined. Take this 60 percent of adults and assume that each has an average of two or three children. These children go on to establish their own adult households based on the lifestyles and philosophies they were raised with (an overweight lifestyle), and then these children each have two or three children of their own. In a few generations the statistics for America will be devastating. In all probability the percentage of obese Americans will reach approximately 80 percent by the next century. We won't have to worry about foreign powers or terrorism destroying this country. Like hungry termites in a piece of rotting driftwood, we will eat and lounge ourselves to oblivion.

Hand-Me-Down Eating

The Keely house is home to Cher, her mother, Celia, and Cher's two girls, Kate and Kelsey. Grandma Celia has been grossly overweight for most of her adult life. Now in her late fifties, Celia must use a walker to get around. She suffers from a variety of chronic illnesses, such as diabetes, asthma, and gout. Although Grandma Celia has great difficulty getting around, she does all the cooking for the family. Raised in the South, Celia learned her cooking skills primarily from her own grandmother, Jesse. Stop and think about this cycle. Kate and Kelsey are growing up on a diet whose roots are *at least* four generations old. Their diet passes through their mom's generation (she doesn't cook) and is determined by their grandmother (Celia), who learned not from her mother (generation number three in this chain) but from *her* grandmother, the fourth generation from Kate and Kelsey. Four generations in time spans at least one hundred years! The tastes, the varieties of food, the nutritional content of their food, and even the presentation of the foods that the 2003 Keely household eats is at least one hundred years old. This cycle is called "hand-me-down eating." It would also not be hard to imagine that one hundred years ago, the Keelys' ancestors ate based on this same cycle of hand-me-down eating inherited from their grandparents, and so on.

This cycle of hand-me-down eating is very well entrenched in families. Just consider how we are all raised. Whether you come from a traditional nuclear family (two birth parents who stay together and raise their own children in one household) or a family that is not so traditional, we all develop our tastes from the environment surrounding us and influencing us from birth. Remember that about five out of every seven adults children see are obese. The adults in control of our young lives determine what we eat in our lives until we take over. Remember Jack's plight? Think about it: Who chose the first solid food that entered your mouth? And what was that choice? Who decided that a fresh-baked chocolate-chip cookie was a special treat to get all excited about? The adults around us did as they excitedly said, "Mmmm... what smells so good in that oven?" and smiled and licked their chops. Did they say the same thing about a head of cauliflower steaming on top of the stove? Of course not, yet both foods give off distinctive odors that fill the house. Now consider that these subliminal messages about eating, our tastes, and our choices are repeated in the home over and over for years. It would seem as if this cycle of hand-me-down eating is impossible to break.

Breaking Down the Fortress of Fat

As if the overt and covert influences of food choices are not enough to lock in the practice of hand-me-down eating, you must add on a family's parenting skills, discipline, and health practices. You are then facing a cultural phenomenon that seems to be impervious to change. How can we break out of this cycle when just twenty years ago pediatricians still believed that a healthy baby was a husky baby? Common medical practice was so innocent of nutritional factors that most doctors relied on the simple correlation that a healthy, thriving baby weighs more than a sickly, at-risk baby. This same logic was applied to pregnancy. Obstetricians advised pregnant women to gain large amounts of weight, instilling in the mother's mind that weight gain and baby's success go hand in hand. We can even mix in here a parent's self-esteem gleaned from these same forces influencing a family. Raise a fat baby and you have a happy baby. Raise a fat baby and you have a healthy, strong baby. Fat is equated with strength and power in all the messages that a parent receives. What a world the baby arrives into: Everywhere the baby turns is a pressure to be fat. The common family life of a child builds a fortress of fat that the child cannot escape, and this cycle repeats itself generation after generation.

As if this fortress of fat built by tastes and age-old parenting techniques is not enough, our common disciplining techniques also use food inappropriately to create fat families. A family "treat" is commonly defined as something to eat, and usually that something is sugary, fat laden, and highly caloric. Parents often reward children with desserts or sweets and punish them by taking the sweets away. Custom dictates that desserts are the fun part of meals and special desserts are part of celebrations. Birthday cakes, ice cream, candy, and other sweets have long been the symbols that something special is happening. Just consider what impressions about food these actions implant into the minds of our children. Not feeling good? Reward yourself with something caloric and sweet. Alone, away from home, feeling lonely? Eat something to reward yourself and make you feel good or even remind you of home.

Some people would add several other bricks onto the walls of our fortress of fat. One of these is the fact that a person's taste buds for sweet and salt are some of the earliest to develop, so how can we avoid being rewarded by sweets and other high-calorie foods? A valid question, but recent studies have some good news and bad news about taste buds. The good news is that even though these tastes develop early, it does not mean that parental food choices cannot override these circuits. A child will learn to eat and, yes, even like foods that don't appease these taste buds. Simply giving a baby other food choices will sidestep this early circuitry until the taste buds become more mature and fully developed. The bad news is that parents can easily become vulnerable to the reward of sweet and salty foods to appease the baby's disposition and make parenting less difficult. So even though physiology is important, it still comes down to the family environment in determining how strong the cycle of obesity will become.

We already have all of this internal and external pressure that pushes us to eat poorly, and we haven't mentioned another critical factor that contributes heavily to this endless cycle of obesity—the activity level of most families. It is no secret that families are getting less and less exercise today. The common recreational interests of the majority of families are moving away from physical activity and centering on more sedentary interests. More importantly, the attitudes of society are reinforcing this movement away from physical activity. Social institutions are not valuing the need for physical activity. For example, fewer schools are emphasizing the importance of physical activity. Only 6 percent of all high schools in the United States require a physical education class for students by the time they are seniors in high school. Similarly, sports programs as choices of extracurricular activities available to students are dropping like flies in our schools. As a society, we are creating sedentary families.

The goal of this book is not to get mired in the reasons why we are fat. That would easily fill several volumes. The purpose here is to provide insight into the powerful forces we face to break out of the painful cycle of obesity. This book is about solutions, but those solutions have to take into account the overwhelming task we face when we try to break out of these cycles that compel us to behave in unhealthy ways. This discussion is essential because if we don't attack fat in the same way it takes over our lives, by fighting the battle on the same turf, then our success in breaking out of this cycle will be short-lived, if ever achieved at all.

Many of the common weight loss programs on the market today just address weight loss without addressing lifestyle change. And those programs that do pay lip service to lifestyle change have not typically focused on changes that attack head-on those negative forces that keep us all in the cycle of obesity. At best, programs talk about lifestyle change but try to avoid clashing head-on with the cultural and family structures that pull us into obesity. Other programs speak about lifestyle change in terms of denial and sacrifice. You will see that our lifestyle change incorporates fun and function within the environment one was raised and continues to live.

If this discussion has made it seem like an impossible task, there is hope. Consider the changes we have made as a society with regard to cigarette smoking. In the last decade there has been a profound change in how we attached ourselves to smoking. People now must huddle outside of buildings to indulge in their habit. Smokers are now viewed as outcasts, and the smell of cigarette smoke results in heads turning to make note of the origin of the offense, whereas, a short time ago, cigarette-polluted air would not have raised an eyebrow. As a society, we are saying that cigarette smokers are not the norm. These statements are breaking a cycle of pain that was almost as strongly reinforced in our world as that of obesity. The problem with smoking is that there are fewer tools available to smokers to help them break out of this painful cycle. However, read on and you will discover how to arm your family with powerful tools to end the painful cycle of obesity.

THINGS TO REMEMBER:
- Obesity exists in both genders equally.
- Fourteen percent of all children in the United States are overweight.
- This percentage has tripled since the 1960s.
- Today's overweight children are 20 to 30 percent heavier than they were ten years ago.
- Obesity is a larger social problem than drug abuse.
- Sixty percent of all adults are overweight.
- Two out of every three adults children see are overweight.
- By the next century, 80 percent of Americans could be overweight if the current trends continue.

CHAPTER TWO

Why Are We All Fat?

In Chapter One we described the cycle of obesity and explained how this generational cycle keeps people trapped in a painful struggle. Here we would like to take a microscope and focus it on the family unit to examine how home life becomes tangled in this cycle of obesity.

Psychologists have long recognized eating as one of the two most basic human needs. The other of these basic needs is sex. Considering that our survival urgently depends on eating, eating and food outrank sex as the most important of the basic human drives. Given this primary importance of food and eating to human life, from a psychological standpoint we are heavily influenced to eat and become obsessed with eating to guarantee our survival.

To understand just how intense the psychology of eating is, consider what happens when you need to gasp for a breath of air. Have you ever been swimming underwater and begun to run out of air? Remember how it felt as you panicked to get to the surface? You struggled to get to the surface no matter what price you had to pay to breathe. This same drive exists in us all in regard to the daily need for food. Fortunately, we live in a society where food is plentiful. Because of this abundance, the intensity of this basic drive is not foremost on our minds like experiencing the panic for air as in our example. But be aware that this intense need for food is there underneath the surface and always pushing us, just like the example of gasping for air.

Another important psychological function of food is as a coping mechanism that helps us handle emotional states. We use food to soothe ourselves in times of stress, sadness, despair, loneliness, and loss. Next to denial, emotional eating is the most-used coping mechanism to help us face those emotional states.

In addition to using food to help us during negative life circumstances, we also use food during times of joy and elation. Food is always a focal point in celebrations, and overindulgence of food is commonly expected in celebrations and joyous events.

Eating and our individual psychology are intimately woven together. Our psychological makeup as humans provides a very large push to be fat.

From a sociological perspective food has always played a major role in organizing groups of people. People gathered together because of food, making eating a very powerful social catalyst.

Just like its utility as a psychological coping mechanism, food and eating have traditionally helped people cope with the natural nervousness of gathering together and socializing. It is much easier to meet new people and hold a conversation if food is there to take the complete focus away from facing people and forcing them to interact. In family life especially, eating has become one of the only times that the modern family gathers and communicates. Food has always provided families a common interest and a gathering place.

Pete, a twenty-something computer jockey, laughed heartily as he joked with his officemates. "Ya' know, I've been dating Denise for six years and I've never been through the front door of her parents' house. Come to think of it, I don't even know what their living room furniture looks like."

One of the guys popped in, "After all these years, don't they like you?"

Pete responded with certainty, "Naw, it's not like that. It's just that if you ever want to find Denise's family, all you've got to do is go into their kitchen. You'll find everybody sittin' around. They got this big ole projection TV downstairs in the rec room, but they sit in that kitchen with the little nineteen-incher, drink a soda or a beer, eat chips and dip, and sit on those hard metal chairs. Hell, for as much as they use it, they should just rent out the rest of the house and live between the kitchen and the bedroom."

The irony was that none of the officemates crowded around him found the hilarity in Pete's story. They didn't laugh because many families follow the same pattern as Denise's; they sit around the kitchen table and use this area as the center of the house.

Making the kitchen the center of family activity is an antiquated practice that has its roots in a time when the world was a more primitive place. Families would commonly gather around the kitchen because homes did not have central heating systems. The hearth or fireplace served as both the cooking area and the central heater. The fire burned continuously. When it was time to cook, you cooked. At other times the hearth provided warmth and light by which to read or do other work. The most fascinating part of this primitive living condition is that this behavior has endured into modern times. People still treat the kitchen as if it is the center of the home, and this tendency has very significant consequences on how a family views the importance of food and eating. Obviously, changing these habits can have a positive effect on overeating and weight control.

Using the kitchen as a communal place strongly influences the ways we use food socially. The kitchen, with its handy convenience and strong association to food, contributes to food and drink becoming a social lubricant. Conversation and being with others becomes associated with food from early childhood on in households that make the kitchen the centerpiece of the home. Food can then be used to hide from conversation that may be difficult. After all, you can't talk if your mouth is full. Instead of learning how to cope with stressful conversations, arguments, and social tensions through other means, food becomes the preferred coping mechanism. It then becomes easier to turn to food later in life as a coping mechanism for other stressful situations. It very well may start with this symbolic use of the kitchen as the center of the home.

The typical family uses food socially in other intriguing ways. Food and drink are often given prominence when one family member wants to entertain another family member. How many times did you hear some variation of these statements growing up: "We have to go out and get some goodies for Uncle Frank when he comes over so he will enjoy himself." Or "Oh, Aunt Martha called and she's going to stop over. We better go get some bakery cookies so she can have them with her tea. She'll like that." Do we stop to think what important messages these statements are leaving in the minds of the children within earshot? The mind of the child certainly absorbs the converse of these statements; that is, if we don't do these things, then the visitor will not have as good a time. Translated, the message says the relative is primarily interested in visiting for our goodies and not for our company. In these situations the emphasis is placed on the foods and not on the relationships. This is not a small point. The social sciences consistently point out that people develop social skills by absorbing these lessons in social relations. By being present as events occur, these messages are conveyed to the child. Their meanings are stored in the brain's memory bank. Being witness to such events has a powerful mentoring aspect to it, and that's how our children learn how to be social human beings. Need proof? Watch youngsters play house or actually entertain their own visitors. Parents often delight in how children mimic their own actions and statements. As we learn how to have a new sensibility toward eating, some of this mimicry may now seem sad rather than delightful.

Often in social situations a family may seem to be helpless victims in the face of the powerful cycle of obese living. Families feel guilty if they try to live a healthy lifestyle around extended family members in social situations. A family may feel like they are not being sociable if they try to continue their healthy habits in the face of others.

Let's visit another family under the microscope, this time in a positive light, and learn how strong these social messages can be. The Lopez family often is invited to one of the many social gatherings their large extended family holds on the weekends. These family gatherings presented a huge obstacle in the past to the Lopez's efforts at establishing a healthy lifestyle. Most often the foods presented at these gatherings were items that the Lopez family was now trying to eliminate from their diet. The Lopez family also learned (from the use of the program in this book) that there are no excuses for indulgence in bad foods, no exceptions, no "one time" dispensations to a healthy lifestyle. They have learned that to apply any of these excuses not only erases days of good effort but also sets up the emotional and symbolic messages that can lead back to a negative lifestyle. In response to these family situations, the Lopez family plans out their time at family functions. Let's listen:

"What's Auntie Maria going to serve at Jenny's baptism party, Mom?" Kara asked.

"Well, I bet Auntie Tina made her usual fiesta salad. I'm going to pick out the salami she puts in it and not use that creamy dressing she puts out on the side. That salad has enough flavors that you don't need any dressing. And I love that fruit Jell-O that Aunt Joanne makes. You know, there's nothing but good stuff in there, just Jell-O and fruit. I'm going for both of those for sure," Mom said.

The rest of the car ride to the party became a lively conversation anticipating what foods the Lopez family would eat that afternoon. Sure, it sounded like a conspiracy, but the conversation helped everyone keep to the goal of a healthy lifestyle. In addition, that discussion probably helped curb any chance that any of the Lopez family would depart from their healthy eating habits because it made their actions conscious, preventing automatic behavior that could lead to mistakes that would make them feel guilty later.

Had the Lopez family not planned out their time at the party in this light, fun way, they may have fallen into a trap. Many families eat foods that are grossly unhealthy under these special circumstances. Later in this book you will see how these special incidents can cost a family days of staying on course in living a healthy lifestyle. For example, one afternoon of unhealthy eating could cost a family member 1,500 calories and as much as 100 grams of fat in just one meal in one day.

Families establish very rigid eating traditions that change slowly over generations. You can see from the above examples that family food habits become very predictable. These traditions don't just dictate where families gather or what foods they bring to large family parties; they determine the fundamental way people eat and what foods they choose. These traditions or eating culture of a family may have become established at a time when the dietary needs of the family demanded certain foods to sustain life. Because these habits change so slowly, the family's dietary needs now may not require the same foods they needed a generation ago. The eating habits that were once adequate to maintain a certain lifestyle are now poor habits in today's world where modern work and recreation needs are so different from a generation ago. Presto! This ingrained food culture of the family only serves to push the family members deeper into the painful cycle of obesity.

Why are we fat? Just considering the two most powerful influences on our behavior, our individual psychology and the sociology that surrounds us, we can see how much we are forced into eating patterns that trap us into poor lifestyle choices. Yet, there are other forces in our lives that keep families caught in the cycle of obesity.

Two very important forces to consider are the physiology of the human body and genetic predispositions handed down from our ancestors.

There is no question that every human body is a unique machine. The ability of one person to eat unhealthy foods and not become obese while another struggles daily with his weight while watching carefully what he eats has been a puzzle to explain. We are still learning about the uniqueness of the human body and the tools to help us solve this puzzle. Metabolic rates (the way the body uses energy) and biochemistry play important roles in how one stays fit, and these vary from person to person. Both of these will be discussed further in Chapter Five.

The uniqueness of each individual has been a huge roadblock to ending obesity. Diet and fitness programs generally do not address individual differences; instead, they are written like newspaper horoscopes. They are so general that anyone can apply the techniques offered. But our bodies are so unique that significant success is accomplished only through individual adjustment of these programs. For that reason, these programs have limited success. A person trying to end obesity uses a program that a friend has had success with only to find that the program doesn't give her the same results. This failure drives the person deeper into the cycle of obesity because she now feels that nothing will work for her. She falls into hopelessness and gives up.

Mark and Cathy are young newlyweds who have devoted themselves to a healthy lifestyle of staying fit and eating right. In their second year of marriage, Mark's employer changed insurance carriers, and Mark and Cathy were required to have an insurance examination. Obtaining the results of this insurance exam, Cathy was shocked to find out that her cholesterol level was almost one hundred points higher than Mark's. They eat the same foods, even when away from each other at lunch or other situations, and both exercise the same number of times each week. Cathy was devastated and became so discouraged that she cut back the number of times she exercised weekly and struggles now to fit her workouts into her schedule.

Cathy cannot accept that a number of factors determine that her cholesterol level is different than Mark's even though they eat and exercise the same. Cathy's body is different, and she will have to consider those differences if she wants her cholesterol level to be similar to Mark's.

It is important to understand that every human body is unique. What works for one person may not work for you or your family members!

__The Family Fit Program is specifically designed to accommodate individual differences.__

Also with respect to the physiology of the human body, many people, including weight loss professionals, believe obese individuals do not burn calories as efficiently as non-obese people. This theory is false. Early studies at the University of Michigan, which were confirmed by studies done at Columbia and Rockefeller universities, showed that obese people burn an average of 1,432 kilocalories for each square meter of body surface just to maintain body weight and to keep the body functioning normally. Non-obese people burn 1,341 kilocalories per square meter of body surface to accomplish the same tasks. The difference between the obese and the non-obese is probably because obese individuals need to burn slightly more calories to maintain the extra pounds they carry. So, in fact, obese and non-obese individuals burn off calories at about the same relative rate.

__It is simply not true that obese people are not as good at burning off calories as non-obese people. "I can't burn off calories as fast as everyone else" should not be used as an excuse for obesity.__

Genetics
The role of genetics deserves special attention here. Families cite genetics as the primary reason for being obese.

Liz, Betty, Claire, Mary, and Jane were in their comfort zone huddled together at a baby shower. Debbie, Betty's sister, walked into the banquet room of the restaurant and immediately joined the group.

"You look great! What's your secret?" Claire said to Debbie as soon as she came near the others.

"Following Family Fit, eating right, and being active! Thanks!" Debbie chuckled, knowing that none of them knew what Family Fit meant.

Betty chimed in, "Oh, I wish I could look like you," she said as she stood and pointed at her plump frame, "but I have the same shape as my mom and her mom did. Just like a tree trunk!" Betty didn't skip a beat with her heredity excuse, even in the face of the admiration being thrown at her *older* sister, Debbie, who certainly had the same mom and grandmom.

There is no doubt that genetics set the table for us to be fat. But whether we dine at that table of fat depends on other factors. Research shows that, except in very, very small percentages of the population, we can overcome this genetic code to be obese through proper diet and fitness activity. Yes, your genetics may make it more difficult for you to keep trim as opposed to your neighbor, and you may have areas of your body that will require special attention, but you can prevent the genetic loading from locking you into a lifetime of obesity.

The facts about genetics reveal that in the last forty to fifty years of gene research related to obesity, gross disruption of the five genes now known to be associated with obesity have only caused *rare* cases of human obesity. Researchers conclude that it seems unlikely that major aberrations in individual genes will emerge as the *sole* cause of a person's weight problem. For that reason, the most important aspect of genetic discoveries has been an improved understanding of the way the body regulates itself. That is the notion that the human body struggles to maintain a *body weight set-point*.

> ***Genetic research shows that the body struggles to maintain a body weight set-point.***

Scientists believe the body weight set-point is a genetically inherited level of body weight that is preset for each individual. When the individual attempts to lose or gain weight, the body will try to regulate itself back to this set-point. But scientists agree that this mechanism can be overruled by the way the individual regulates his or her weight.

> ***Scientists agree that obesity is absolutely dependent on the availability of food and its consumption.***

The conclusion is that the current state of genetic research is clouded by the undeniable importance of behavior and environment.

> ***Don't let genetics be your excuse for being fat!***

There is no evidence that shows that genetics will prevent you from looking, feeling, and staying healthy. Stop using the genetics excuse to keep you from doing what you need to do to be healthy. The genetics excuse is simply not true.

The Fear of Eating Disorders

Some families may be hesitant to include the youngest family members in a program that will stress a lifestyle change in eating and that will discuss nutrition, calorie counting, fitness, and the other concepts discussed in this chapter. This reluctance may arise from the fear that the children will develop eating disorders as a result of this new family consciousness. In response to this fear it is important to reiterate that the new family orientation toward food and eating stresses having fun, enjoying food, and educating each other on eating well. These new family attitudes are opposite those held by people who suffer from eating disorders.

Eating disorders are unique mental dysfunctions that have symptoms involving the regulation of food. The *Diagnostic and Statistical Manual of Mental Disorders* classifies these disorders as mental diseases. There are many forms of eating disorders ranging from starving oneself (anorexia) to bingeing and purging (bulimia).

These disorders most commonly develop in teens. They are also more common in girls than boys. The exact causes of these disorders are not specifically known, but they are believed to be multidetermined. Often they start when young people copy the behavior of peers who exhibit or experiment with the symptoms of these disorders. A common psychological purpose of the symptoms is the intense need to have control of one's life in reaction to a parenting style that the young person sees as overcontrolling. It is clear that these disorders are not caused by being concerned about what one eats or by being enthusiastic about fitness. It is perfectly safe for young children to be raised in a home that adheres to the practices and philosophies of this program, which stresses a positive lifestyle. The result will be a healthy, happy lifestyle and not the development of an eating disorder.

THINGS TO REMEMBER:
- Food is the most powerful reinforcement in life.
- Food is a basic coping mechanism.
- Food is a traditional social catalyst.
- Genetics are no excuse for not eating healthy and being physically active.
- The body will struggle to maintain a body weight set-point.
- If children are included in a fitness program, they will not be more likely to develop an eating disorder.

PART II
THE BIG PICTURE

CHAPTER THREE

Preparing for the Program

One of the keys to breaking the family fat curse is preparation before beginning the program. One of the common pitfalls of the popular weight loss programs offered to the public in recent years is the demand that the person(s) jump right in to the program without preparation. Unfortunately, research has shown that without preparation for any new behavior the chances for success are diminished enormously. It is contrary to human endeavor to undertake a new experience without preparation beforehand. Would you enter a triathlon without preparation? Of course not. So why in the world would you begin a program that attempts to change habits that you and your family have had for generations without preparation? Preparation helps us emotionally as well as physically. Get the hint? This chapter is very important to your success.

Preparing for our program takes some doing. The opening two chapters of this book emphasized how the cycle of obesity places a stranglehold on family members as a result of many powerful forces. These forces originated generations ago. It is essential to first understand that these forces exist (Chapter One) and then realize how they operate to keep us fat (Chapter Two). Now you must try to control as many of these forces as possible as you prepare to start our program.

Read this chapter and begin to think about how you can change the forces that prod us to be fat. Start changing these forces in the life of your family. Then read through the whole book and come back to this chapter before you start the program. Remember, this preparation is essential to success and a key reason why other programs fail. Be a good scout and be prepared.

Now we are going to examine those major forces mentioned in the first two chapters and explain ways in which you can better control their influence on you and your family members.

Generational Forces

Give your immediate family members this book so they can read about these forces themselves. Everyone in your household should be familiar with how the family lifestyle is going to change. To do this you have to take charge. "Here's something we are going to do for ourselves." One family member will have to be the leader for the others if this program is to be a success. Present this program as a "done deal" to the family. After all, if there were any other health need that your family required, you would put it into action without a democratic process. You would just do it. Why should the number one health concern across the country be treated any differently?

Consider how a family handles childhood vaccinations. You listen to good, sound medical advice that taking this preventive action will improve the lives of your children. You make the decision to go through this series of inoculations and take this leadership in your family. If you left it up to a democratic process, let's say a vote, would the youngsters vote to subject themselves to this painful experience? Probably not. *You* decide that it is in the best interests of the family to include this preventive action in your lifestyle.

The key to adult leadership when you have tiny ones in your immediate family is not to exclude them from knowing about the changes that will take place around them. As you read on in the book, you will see how this program incorporates *every* generation. It is just as important for the little ones to know what is happening as it is for the older ones. Instead of expecting the little ones to read this book, talk to them about what you are learning from it. Lead family discussions about the program the family will be starting. Communication here is the key. This is the best preparation for change. Let's go back to our example of the vaccinations. The best preparation you can give your children for getting shots is to communicate with them about what will happen. Talk to them and guide them into picturing the procedure, how it will feel, how long it will last. We know that the source of all fear arises from the unknown. If you let this experience, or any experience, come at your family without preparation, then the fear is heightened and the experience fails. This is a guiding principle of our program.

Success is enhanced by good preparation.

Preparation dispels fears of the unknown before they arise. What will we eat? How will it taste? What will we do? These are all natural questions that are certain to arise when trying to implement new behaviors. Let them know, explain how it will taste and feel, help them picture the experience. Be very detailed in your descriptions. Your assurances will guide the family into this new lifestyle.

When you take this leadership with the program, make sure you include every extended family member who is going to influence your life, not just the immediate family. Give this book to extended family members as a gift. Let them know, "This is the manual my family and I are following. Whether you join in this program is up to you. That would be great, but I wanted you to have this to know what we're going through. So if I don't eat the same way or don't seem like I appreciate your hospitality, it's really not that at all. We're just trying to live differently. We love visiting and being with you."

You can certainly change this script and make it longer or shorter to explain what you're doing. No matter how you say it, give them a copy of the book and they will understand better and hopefully support you.

Certainly, some of the most difficult extended family members to face with your new lifestyle will be those family members who influenced you as you were growing up. Mothers, fathers, grandparents, older siblings, aunts, and uncles are some of the hardest people to face when you are trying to be different. What's the key to coping with these people as you practice your new lifestyle? The key can be stated in one word:

Resolve

They may criticize, joke, or even insult you, but if you believe in your program and the well-being of your family, then nothing these negative people can say will have any effect on what you and your family are accomplishing. The more you confidently maintain your resolve, the more these potential critics will melt away.

Aunt Ann was an old-school, meat-and-potatoes cook who was raised to immediately bring out loads of traditional ethnic foods for visitors. She was a hard-drinking chain smoker well into her sixties and always had a snappy, smart-aleck remark when a family member mentioned any of her negative behaviors. Aunt Ann's niece, Beth, and her family loved Aunt Ann's basic goodness and kindness but found it increasingly hard to visit Aunt Ann as they changed their eating habits. It wasn't just the presentation of food; the visit became a tug-of-war between differing lifestyles. Aunt Ann was always defensive and sarcastic as the visits wore on and the food she served just sat there. To their credit, even though Aunt Ann always intimidated them, Beth and her family would explain that they didn't eat those foods anymore. This bounty of foods went untouched visit after visit until one day, in her usual sweet voice, Aunt Ann invited Beth and the family over and eagerly added, "I'm going to make something you and the kids will like. I found a recipe for a low-calorie, low-fat cheesecake, and I can't wait to try it." Needless to say, after countless visits full of negative food experiences at Aunt Ann's, Beth was astounded to hear Aunt Ann change her stripes. Beth always came away from visiting Aunt Ann thinking that her family's positive lifestyle was leaving a bitter taste in Aunt Ann's mouth. The resolve and confidence shown by Beth and the family wore down Aunt Ann's negativity.

Cleaning House

In the first step of preparation we have tried to control as much as possible the generational forces that can interfere with our program. Next we have to control our immediate environment by "cleaning house."

In cleaning house we start with the obvious place—the refrigerator. Without hesitation, without excuses or rationalizations, remove every item that is high calorie and has a high saturated fat content. *Do not* excuse an item with rationalizations such as: This is a waste of money. I'll save this for company. I'll wait and give this to a charity. Someday I may be able to eat/drink this again. This is for the kids. This is for the kids' friends when they come over. Or any variation of these or any other excuse you may make. Just get rid of these items now.

The worst items are butter, mayonnaise, margarine, whole milk, cream, cheese, ice cream, ice cream bars, frozen fried foods, leftover fried foods, restaurant leftovers, luncheon meats (except for light lean beef, light turkey, light ham, and light chicken), condiments that are high in calories and fat, sodas, and salad dressings (except for light, low-fat salad dressings), particularly mayonnaise-based salad dressings. Throw them all out now.

Next, move over to the pantry, shelves, and cupboard. Do the same thing. Throw out any high-calorie and high-fat food item. No excuses. There should be no such thing in your cabinets as cookies, candy, regular peanut butter, macaroni and cheese mix, canned chili, canned corned beef hash, canned spaghetti, boxed au gratin potatoes, boxes of snack foods, high-caloric cereals, and boxes of quick meal preparations. Throw out any dry goods that are high in fat and in calories. Yes, do this now!

Do not ever bring these foods back into your house again. It creates a dramatic effect to bring together the family to help in this housecleaning. By doing so the family sees you mean business, and they learn important nutritional lessons as you explain why these things need to be thrown out. You can turn this task into a game of scavenger hunt for all the "bad" foods that have to be junked. Youngsters will delight in the act of throwing things away. It will seem so forbidden to them that they may enjoy feeling as if they are doing something "bad" themselves. If they do join in, explain to young people what this action is all about. Capitalize on this golden teaching moment. On the next page is a worksheet called *Family Planner—Food List*. It is provided to stimulate your family into helping with cleaning the house of unhealthy foods. Sit down with your family and present this worksheet like a game; think of all the foods that keep you fat and then brainstorm substitutes. Or you could post the Food List in a very conspicuous spot in the house, on the refrigerator for example, and let the family write in their suggestions. Even if you use the Food List like a game one evening, don't let it be a one-time exercise. Feel free to make copies of the Food List. Post them in more than one place in the house. This will allow the family to think of new ideas continuously, and it will use this tool to its fullest. It can be great fun. Try it.

FAMILY PLANNER—FOOD LIST

Unhealthy Food Item   Healthy Food Item

Now, here comes a very important mind-set in preparing for the program. You are not denying yourself or your family from ever eating and enjoying any type of food. This program is not about denying you anything. It is about enjoyment of life and a healthy, positive, fun lifestyle. All of these items that you are discarding can be replaced with alternatives that taste just as good and are better for you and your family. This statement couldn't have been made as recently as five years ago, but food science has progressed to the point that all unhealthy foods have a healthier substitute.

In Chapter Five we present a chart that provides one-to-one substitutions for the common foods that keep us in the cycle of obesity. These alternatives taste, feel, and look the same as the Neanderthal foods we have been consuming for hundreds of years. Don't sabotage this program with excuses such as, "This doesn't taste the same made this way." These statements are mind games that will take you back to a lifestyle that will propel you into the cycle of obesity.

If you are old enough to remember when diet sodas were first developed, this experience will help you develop a better mind-set about changing your food choices. When diet sodas were first developed, many consumers exclaimed, "This has a chemical taste!" As a result many people rejected diet sodas as a substitute for regular soda. Today, diet sodas are widely popular and people seldom complain about their taste. Healthier foods that are substitutes for unhealthy foods can follow the same evolution in your home if you allow it to happen. In fact, most of the healthier food substitutes taste much closer to the traditional food than diet sodas tasted to regular soda. Today, the transition should be even smoother in substituting foods. Most often families don't stick with the healthier food substitutes because a family member complains. Instead of the adult family leader being patient and sticking with the change, he immediately caves into the complaint, no matter how minor, and changes back to the unhealthy traditional food. It is time to take a stand on this issue as a family and learn to accommodate a healthier eating lifestyle. Make this healthy eating transition when you clean house in preparation for this program and don't turn back.

Comb the Territory

Although unhealthy foods are a huge contributor to our family cycle of obesity, unhealthy foods are not the only problems in our households. When cleaning house, we have to examine the symbols and messages all around us that perpetuate the obese family lifestyle.

In Chapter Two we talked about a young lady's family who sat around the kitchen table constantly. This is a good example of how an unhealthy message about the importance of eating and food becomes a family habit. This is precisely the type of message you will need to examine as you take the next step in cleaning house, called "combing the territory."

First, look at the habits of your family that contribute to overeating and lack of activity. List the habit and think immediately of the ways you can change that habit and what new habit you can put in its place.

Next, look at *things* you have around the house that keep you fat. Like the food game we first discussed in cleaning house, you can make a family game of both of these activities. To help, on the following pages there are more Family Planners—one for Habits and one for Things. Use them just like the Family Planner—Food List provided previously. Have fun filling these out with the family.

Sitting at the kitchen table is a good example for the Habits chart. If your family treats the kitchen table as the center of your home, think of how to change that activity. Then replace that bad habit with a new one. Maybe you can meet in the family room or living room instead.

FAMILY PLANNER—HABITS

Unhealthy Habit	How It Has Changed	Healthy New Habit
_____	_____	_____
_____	_____	_____
_____	_____	_____
_____	_____	_____
_____	_____	_____
_____	_____	_____
_____	_____	_____
_____	_____	_____
_____	_____	_____
_____	_____	_____
_____	_____	_____
_____	_____	_____
_____	_____	_____
_____	_____	_____
_____	_____	_____
_____	_____	_____
_____	_____	_____
_____	_____	_____
_____	_____	_____
_____	_____	_____

FAMILY PLANNER—THINGS

Fat Thing   New Thing   How to Replace It
_____   _____   _____
_____   _____   _____
_____   _____   _____
_____   _____   _____
_____   _____   _____
_____   _____   _____
_____   _____   _____
_____   _____   _____
_____   _____   _____
_____   _____   _____
_____   _____   _____
_____   _____   _____
_____   _____   _____
_____   _____   _____
_____   _____   _____
_____   _____   _____
_____   _____   _____

Let's take an in-depth look at some objects that promote unhealthy habits. A subtle area to examine is the magazines to which you subscribe. The reading materials that sit around our houses not only symbolize our tastes but also give off subliminal messages to everyone in the house. Think about it. If the only magazines you have around the house are television guides, video game aficionado magazines, food magazines, or entertainment magazines, these choices indicate your preference for passive entertainment and traditional eating. And having these magazines around the house sends a message to all family members that this is your philosophy of life. These are the things that are important. If you want to change from an unhealthy to a healthy lifestyle and end the cycle of obesity, then you should change the statements that these colorful, inviting magazines give off by lying around the house like miniposters for a sedentary, gluttonous lifestyle. They stare everyone in the face on a daily basis. Begin a subscription to at least one fitness or health magazine. Make sure you leave these magazines out prominently. Consider canceling magazines that advertise and promote the unhealthy lifestyle your family is leaving behind.

Look for other objects around the house. Is there a television in every room? Is your home set up to invite family members to hide in their little enclaves and retreat from interaction with others? Do you have a place where you can have a family meal, or do people eat alone, isolated from the rest of the family? If this is the case, overeating and hoarding food are easier. In addition, accountability is lessened. When trying to establish a new lifestyle, eating together establishes accountability toward one another.

Preparing Meals
How we obtain our food is an important issue for this program and typically not addressed by other programs. We can easily get into

unhealthy habits in the way we gather our meals. In this preparation take a look at how family members get their food at each meal. Is breakfast a free-for-all where people grab whatever they feel like? If so, then accountability for following the program can get lost. Do family members buy their own food at lunch? How can they be expected to follow the program if they are left with no support? Obviously, this is particularly true with the youngest family members. Certainly, we can't be expected to follow each family member around throughout the day and ensure that everyone is making healthy choices, but the temptation to depart from the program can be decreased tremendously if family members are restricted from unhealthy choices. At lunch this may mean brown bagging and restricting the amount of money one carries around to resist buying unhealthy supplements to the brown-bag lunch.

In Chapter Six you will read how family members become self-motivated and instinctively follow the program guidelines with the motivational techniques discussed there. But as you set up the preparations for the program with the techniques and thinking outlined here, you will see how many of these preparations foster motivation and adherence to the program in a very powerful way. What is suggested here are ways to develop new habits that will have intrinsic self-motivation. It is much like building a house; the better you have built the foundation, the stronger the rest of the house will be.

Dinner habits follow this same thought. If you allow your family members to eat on their own, isolated from the rest of the family, the motivation to keep with the program can be shattered. Try to eat as a family at dinner as much as possible. Even if you have to change the dinner hour to later, try to accommodate the entire family at dinner. If one family member on a rare occasion must eat separately, then make sure he or she is eating exactly the same as the rest of the family that evening. Prepare his or her dinner with the others and set it aside.

Meals in this program provide a built-in system of checks and balances. As a result, eating habits in the manner outlined above are very important in making the other steps of the program as effective as possible. Changing our mealtime habits is very effective housecleaning.

Watch Your Mouth

We need to prepare our mouths not only to eat in a new way but to speak in a new way. Those of us caught in the cycle of obesity *talk fat*. We have grown up talking about food, eating, and activity in an unhealthy way. Our eyes light up at the possibility of a special dessert. Certain foods bring big smiles to our faces, and we use words to describe them such as "Oh…what a treat!" or "Let's live a little!" or "Let's celebrate!"

Speech and body language are powerful, subliminal influences on our behavior and on everyone around us. It will take careful thought to change the way you speak in the presence of your family as you prepare to change your lifestyle. If you do not speak the language of healthy living, your family members can get the subtle message that the entire endeavor is just some kind of a phase you are going through that will pass. They will get the message that you are not serious about the changes you are talking about. If you change the way you speak, then your language can be a powerful tool that will keep you on track with the program goals.

Talking about alcohol abuse is a good example of how language can subtly, unconsciously sabotage our efforts to lead a healthy lifestyle. How many times have you been to a family party where a relative drinks too much and becomes less inhibited, more jovial, and downright silly? We try to set a good example for our family and discuss proper use of alcohol, but we inadvertently talk about the drunk relative something like this: *(laughing)* "Wasn't Uncle Charlie hilarious when he stood on the table and tried to do the twist? When he fell off, the whole house shook. Wow—talk about your big bang theory. That guy was so drunk, I don't think he'll remember a thing." (*more laughing*)

Talking like this conveys that it is fun and funny to drink too much. It also conveys that you support Uncle Charlie's behavior. In reality, it is sad that this man drank that much. And it is sad that the other guests at the party enabled him to act in that manner. Laughing at his behavior only supports a negative lifestyle.

We talk the same way about overeating: (*laughing*) "Wow! Did you see Aunt Edie pound down those cookies?" Laughing about a behavior like this makes the statement that it is fun to eat something unhealthy and even more fun when you eat to excess or gluttony. So, children, if you want to make us all laugh, shove cookies down your throat just like Aunt Edie. Watch how you talk about others' behavior when they are being unhealthy in front of your family.

A common time where we get caught talking supportively about unhealthy behavior without realizing it is when we are communicating with our older relatives. It is very common to forgive their unhealthy practices and speak as if we agree with their statements about food, eating, or activity. Let's consider an example. Grandpa Byrnes, a short, round man of five feet six inches and nearly three hundred pounds, proclaims, "Hey, I've been eating Grandma Byrnes's Boston cream pie once a week for years, and I'm as healthy as a horse. There's nothing wrong with eating some pie every couple of days. You know what's wrong nowadays? Everybody wants to be too skinny. That's dumb."

Quite often an older family member makes such a statement, and we remain silent as the rest of our family listens. Not speaking up symbolizes agreement, but you do not wish to speak disrespectfully to an older person. You don't have to answer Grandpa Byrnes's proclamation by pointing out that he is not only as healthy as a horse but also as large as a horse, thanks to those pies. A delicate response, yet one that conveys to your family that Grandpa's thinking is wrong, can go something like this: "Grandpa, there's no doubt that Grandma's pies taste good and that you enjoy them, but we want to lose weight and stay fit. Those pies have too many calories for us." Now Grandpa may still grumble, but you have made your point for the rest of the family to hear without being disrespectful.

A few classic comments older family members make are land mines that explode right in front of our efforts to keep our families on track with a healthy lifestyle. These sayings have been so common in families for generations that they deserve singling out. These are phrases such as "Clean your plate," "You have to eat more meat," "There's plenty, have another helping," "Fill that plate," "You can't have anything to drink until you eat everything on your plate," "You're going to make the cook feel bad if you don't eat," and the all-time, ageless classic, "There are people starving in China. Now don't complain and eat everything put in front of you."

Anytime any of these or similar sayings are inflicted upon your family, it is time for an adult to step in and correct this thinking. If these incidents, no matter how isolated, keep dangling in front of a family, we have no control over how the family will react and what they will absorb from these actions. They must be overridden.

Learn a New Language

Language has such a powerful influence on people that it is important to practice and think about how we talk in preparation for starting the program. On the next page there is a Family Planner for speech. As with the other Family Planners, they make great starting points for a fun exercise with the family. Sit down with this one and think about how each family member talks about food and physical activity in unhealthy ways. Here's a big tip: It is common to talk about unhealthy foods as if they are forbidden. If we attach such a mystique to them, it makes them seem special. Do that and you will make family members curious about them. Family members, particularly younger ones, will be more motivated to try them. This same relationship is true for unhealthy places to eat, such as most fast-food restaurants. The best way to talk about unhealthy foods and unhealthy places is to be indifferent about them. They should just not matter in your family's life. These things are no big deal.

For example, Joe and Dianne were walking down the hallway of their apartment building one morning. Dianne smelled frying bacon coming from a neighbor's apartment. As she recognized the scent, she exclaimed, "Bacon! Oh, man, I wish I could eat that. It has been so long."

Dianne's words and expression made this unhealthy food seem as if it were special, something rare. This is a very bad message. Words and expressions like this stir up all kinds of emotional reaction to this food and create a want or need for it as if it were forbidden fruit.

FAMILY PLANNER—HOW WE TALK

Unhealthy Ways We Talk   New Healthy Ways We Talk

Forward Thinking

A very important skill that will prepare you and your family for success in this program is thinking ahead when situations are coming that could potentially derail your program.

Family parties, work-related gatherings, dining out at restaurants—these are all occasions that will challenge the healthy habits learned in this book. Planning ahead is the best method for handling these situations. Anticipate what foods will be served and plan your strategy. Involve the whole family in this planning if they are also going to attend. Most of us have been at dozens of these events. There are very few food surprises, yet we often act as if each event is the first time we have seen, let alone tasted, these foods. Plan what you are going to eat, and look for it when you are there. Or don't eat at all. Just plan to eat before or after the event. All of this sounds outrageous but, after all, why are we at the event? If it is a relative's function, it should be to visit, not to eat.

Sadly, in many families it appears as if the focus has been turned around. Family parties get judged by the quantity and quality of the food served and not by the celebration. Concentrate on the visiting and socializing and not the eating.

If it is a work-related function, you are there for business, not for eating. Concentrate on your business-related relationships, ignore the food—be indifferent to it.

If you or just one family member is going to attend an outside event, a great way to keep family members on track with the program is to make sure you "check in" with that person afterward. Ask how he handled it. What did he eat? How did he avoid the "bad stuff"? Smile and support his efforts. Congratulate him on his commitment. This is a great way to help each family member stay with the program goals.

Certainly, one of the common unhealthy side effects of these outside events is that they raise our stress levels, and we eat unhealthily in response. Food can still be used as a coping mechanism at these affairs, but consider what foods you are fingering as you meet your new regional coordinator for the first time. And when this new regional coordinator asks you the $65,000 question you wanted to avoid, just make sure that the broccoli floret you shove in your mouth isn't dipped in the Roquefort dressing. Just shove the broccoli in your mouth and shut up. The question will go away.

Stress at these outside events doesn't always develop because the event is negative. Stress also comes from positive events, and for generations we have coped with it in the same manner as the stress generated from negative events. We just have not been very conscious of this positive stress, so our use of food in these situations has been even more insidious. Unhealthy eating at a celebration can really sneak up on you; before you know it, you have ruined several days of a great new lifestyle. Be careful of family celebrations and other happy events. They can make us veer off the track just as easily as negative events, maybe even more so because they creep up on us like this. Be prepared.

Age

You may have this question at this point: "With all this talk of family participation, at what age should a family member be included in this program?" This question is actually a two-part question in disguise because you want to know at what age family members should be included and at what age family members should stop participating in the program. Even though it's a two-part question, there is a straightforward, one-part answer: People of all ages can participate in this program, from birth to death. This age range is so wide because, unlike other programs, this program does not demand you eat specific foods, do specific activities, or follow specific motivation techniques. Instead, it calls for nutrition tailored to the needs of each family, a choice of activities that please individual families, and motivation techniques most effective for the success of each specific family using this program. Most importantly, you can include infants in your family program from the start. In the past our babies have been born into a society that surrounds them with messages to be fat and lethargic. It is now time to introduce them to a world that stresses healthy eating and fitness.

THINGS TO REMEMBER:
- Prepare before jumping into this program.
- Clean the house of negative foods and messages.
- Fill out the Family Planners.
- Don't talk fat.
- Think ahead when special events or celebrations arise.
- Take control of your lifestyle.
- Children should be a part of this program from birth.

CHAPTER FOUR

The Program Overview: The Three Pillars

Now let's outline the program itself and how it works. We call it the *Family Fit Program*. In the program, all you have to remember is the number *three*. There are three ways you have to follow this program. Family Fit has three elements, called *pillars*, which hold up the program. Each pillar has three tools, or fortifiers, that help it succeed.

The three pillars of the program are
    1) Diet and Nutrition
    2) Activity
    3) Motivation

These pillars are interconnected. One cannot work without the other. It is important to emphasize that each of these pillars is as essential to your success as the others. This emphasis is important because other programs focus on one of these elements and, at best, give a token mention to one of the others. Dieting is typically the main focus. This is a fundamental mistake and a leading cause of why people have not been successful at breaking the generational cycle of obesity.

All of the elements of this program, the three pillars and their fortifiers, are constituted in a unique way. Take an element away or diminish the importance of an element, and you do not have Family Fit any longer. The latest obesity research shows that this approach is the most successful in ending the cycle of obesity that has been harming our families for generations. Successful weight control *will not* take place without all of the pillars and fortifiers: a healthy diet, an active lifestyle, and continual motivation to stay healthy.

No doubt you gained a sense of the uniqueness of this program from reading the first three chapters. The Family Fit Program addresses *all* the forces that contribute to generational obesity and stops them from compelling people to fail. The Family Fit Program is not a difficult program to follow, but it is essential to follow all the elements equally as well as the preparation.

Another key aspect to the Family Fit Program is *fun*. The guiding philosophy of the program is:

If it's not fun, you're done!

To make it fun and easy all you still have to remember is the number *three*. Each of the three basic pillars, diet and nutrition, activity, and motivation, has three basic fortifiers to help you succeed. Finally, it takes only three weeks for you to realize your success. So everything in the program is about threes.

As your family interconnects through this program, you will create a strong, impenetrable bond. The strength of the family unit is how it interconnects to change a lifestyle in spite of generations-old forces of unhealthy thinking and habits. This family unit can make these changes because of the tight bond formed. You can now fully appreciate how these past straight-line approaches are too limited to end generations of obese habits.

Avoid the "Flatline" Approach

Tara, Ken, and their four children sadly illustrate how weak the flatline approach (not keeping diet and nutrition, motivation, and activity equally balanced in your life) is to fighting generational obesity. Tara and Ken are committed to fighting the obesity that plagued both sets of their parents. To fight their tendency to be overweight they both work hard to watch what they eat. They also strictly watch what their children eat. Unfortunately, they have only been exposed to a flatline approach. They bought a diet book written by a movie star, and they follow the eating guidelines of this book. These directions guide them to healthy eating. But this restrictive eating method is the only thing they are doing toward leading a healthy lifestyle to prevent obesity in their family. One of the primary examples of their flatline lifestyle is their failure to control the influence of extended family members. Every Sunday they participate in a large family gathering at Ken's parents' house. Everyone comes. Almost each Sunday Ken's mom cooks her "famous" fried chicken with all the fixings. Several aunts and uncles bring baked goods. Everyone has a good time. Ken and Tara do not make any effort to curb their children's or their own appetite for all the traditional goodies spread out before them. To make matters worse,

Ken and Tara talk up these visits throughout the week. When they speak of the weekly food fest, their body language is excited and animated. They clearly convey that this is a special event that they greatly look forward to during the workweek. Their four children receive the message that this event is more important than what the family accomplishes throughout the week.

Let's take a closer look at what this family could do if they were following the Family Fit Program. Their first fundamental mistake is not treating Sunday as if it were just another day in their program of eating right. They also need to communicate with Grandma that they are eating differently. This communication pulls Grandma into the new lifestyle that Tara and Ken are trying to create.

Again, many people find this discussion with a person of an older generation very difficult or even forbidden. The following model is a good tool for mustering the courage to have this discussion: If you or a family member had to go on a special, doctor-prescribed diet because of an illness, you would easily talk to Grandma about these new special needs, and Grandma would probably be understanding and supportive. At the next Sunday gathering Grandma would probably have special foods or special preparations for dishes that she serves.

This same relationship can and should be used when discussing obesity with the older generation. Obesity is just as serious a health concern as any other illness. When discussing your health needs concerning obesity, have the same conviction and seriousness as you would any of these other illnesses. This commitment will make these discussions with extended family members easier. You may be surprised by how they react when you show this attitude. Deep-fried chicken becomes baked skinless chicken breasts with Grandma's special seasonings. Buttery mashed potatoes are now made without butter and whole milk. Cucumber salad made with mayonnaise now becomes a cucumber salad with sweet-and-sour vinaigrette. A fruit pie can easily be made without loads of sugar and butter.

Involving Grandma in your commitment to healthy eating places her in a more active, meaningful position in the family. Centering your concerns on the grandchildren is another powerful tool in getting grandparents to cooperate with the Family Fit Program. Grandparents love nothing more than to nurture their grandchildren. If you place the health of the grandchildren at the forefront of any talk about health or a new lifestyle, you will increase the cooperation from this generation. Along those same lines, consider that a huge problem the aged face is the lack of meaningful positions in the modern family. Pulling grandparents into the Family Fit Program gives them an important role in the family. Plenty of evidence suggests that getting cooperation from older generations and extended family will not be as difficult as you may think. This issue will be discussed at greater length later in the book.

But you may still protest, "This won't work with my grandparents. You don't know how they are!" These techniques will work with any generation. Look at how families have changed their behavior toward smoking. Remember how many relatives would smoke indoors in front of the children? This very powerful habit has changed dramatically in a short time period. If we can change how people act around this addictive behavior, we can change how they react around eating.

A technique you can use to change people's eating behaviors is to take control of situations at the homes of extended family members. Here's an example. You have discussed your new eating habits with a relative, but when you arrive at her home for a family party, she doesn't serve foods that your family will eat. Take control of the situation by altering the foods presented to meet your new needs. Some of these steps are easy to do, and many will not call any attention to what you are doing or cause embarrassment for the cook.

For example, if you take the skin off deep-fried chicken or fish, it becomes a much healthier dish. Ask what ingredients are in the side dishes presented. If they are made with ingredients that boost their calorie and fat content, choose other items being served. If a dish has some ingredients that can be simply removed, do so; the rest of the dish may be healthy enough to fit into your Family Fit Program. A prime example here is cheese. Quite often people make a relatively healthy dish and then top it with cheese or cheese sauce. Get it out of there. Give your family whispered messages to avoid dishes you know are not healthy. You will be delighted to see youngsters copy this behavior at other family get-togethers when they whisper to you, "Watch out for the slaw…it's deadly."

Another corrective approach to these family events is to anticipate a relative's stubbornness to change for your family and bring along your own side dishes, such as a fresh fruit salad. No one will notice that you did this in reaction to how they eat. The guests will assume you brought the dish just as everyone else brought something to add to the meal. If Tara and Ken would try one of these corrective approaches to the Sunday gathering not only would the children get a great positive message, but also they could possibly generate some curiosity from others, and it could be a learning experience for all.

This true family story illustrates a fundamental principle of the Family Fit Program:

Become powerful in your world.

Keeping the three pillars of the program operating in your family keeps your family powerful in their world. To maintain this strength within the program, each pillar is bolstered by three fortifiers. Remember, everything you need to know in the program is in threes. Each fortifier keeps the pillar strong and powerful in the face of all those generational forces that traditionally would plunge a family member back into the painful cycle of obesity.

The Diet/Nutrition pillar is fortified by the New Habits, Cleanup, and Forward Thinking tools. The Activity pillar is fortified by the Individual Goals, Family Goals, and Generational Goals tools. The Motivation pillar is fortified by the Your Surroundings, Self-Motivation, and Person-to-Person Motivation tools.

In chapters to come each of the pillars will be discussed more thoroughly. The role of these fortifiers in strengthening the Family Fit element will also be discussed. You may have noticed that several of these fortifiers have already been introduced in the book to help describe how the cycle of obesity traditionally traps family members.

Along with fortifiers, another way to become more powerful is to be in control of your world. To do that the Family Fit Program takes the three pillars, Diet/Nutrition, Activity, and Motivation, and provides the family with a daily outline that adds them to a family's lifestyle. This outline is called the Family Day Planner.

Note that this Family Day Planner is not called a schedule and is not presented in blocks of time. Families today lead complex, full lives. The modern family is also defined differently than it was even ten years ago. Single-parent families, divorced families, joint-custody families, and blended families have to accommodate many generations of family members or family members who move in and out of the family environment.

To presume that a family can follow some hour-by-hour plan based on the stereotypical family is ridiculous. Today's family would reject our program at first glance because they would look at such a rigidly defined schedule and deem it unworkable in their household. Or a family may want to try a program so desperately that they attempt to keep up with an hour-by-hour formula only to give up quickly because the time demands cannot be applied to their individual situation. This latter scenario is often the failure of many exercise programs. These programs present a set of exercises and a schedule that is geared to such a broad range of abilities that the unique needs of the individual become lost. These programs fail to see that this uniqueness in individuals is more commonplace than their broad-brush approach.

Here in the Family Fit Program the uniqueness of families is built into the program. The Family Day Planner outlines segments of the day rather than hours, and it can be adjusted to fit a family's demands. For example, a second Day Planner is presented that changes the activity segment from morning to evening. Finally, blank Day Planner Worksheets, one for each week of the program, are given for families to fill out on their own. To do so, keep the segments as presented but juggle them to meet the individual needs of your family. A prime example of this ability to juggle would be in a family where one parent works a graveyard shift. Even with this graveyard schedule, the Day Planner can be rearranged to fit this family. As you can see by this variation in family life, an hour-by-hour schedule just cannot work as a template.

Let's take a closer look at the Day Planners. The Family Fit Program takes just three weeks to achieve success. Notice that we have changed the way the week is normally presented. Most calendars start the week on Sunday. To be successful for your family, Family Fit starts the week on Saturday. Beginning the week on Saturday provides more time for family involvement. The program starts on Saturday and then voila! The next day, Sunday, allows the family to continue with the momentum built up in their first day of participation. Then we head into Monday, a typical back-to-school, back-to-work day. You'll notice on the Day Planner that Monday can be a day off from the fitness activity segment of the Family Fit Program.

This is very significant. The mind-set of many people starting new self-improvement programs is often, "I'll start on Monday." This attitude is often the first step to failure. The I'll-start-on-Monday attitude has long been chronicled by weight loss experts as a common deferral for starting a new health regime. We all know that Monday is often the most intensely busy and unpredictable day of the week. You try to start on Monday, but something unexpected comes up and you don't complete your goals, so the program doesn't get off the ground. Now you push the start to another Monday, and that Monday gets aborted like the first Monday, and so on and so on. This is called the Monday–Monday excuse. You'll quickly find yourself back in the cycle of obesity.

In the Family Fit Program, the Monday–Monday excuse is sidetracked. Family Fit takes the fitness activity segment out of Monday so that Mondays are not a burden. Incidentally, you can't blame Family Fit for a bad Monday because it can be your activity rest day. In fact, Family Fit may just have you looking forward to Mondays. This again can be a failure of other programs. You add to a Monday the start of a new program, you have a bad Monday, and this creates a negative reinforcement for your new program. So what gets abandoned, particularly on the next Monday? Your brand-new program: You give it up and become convinced that programs just don't work for you.

Breaking It Down

Returning to the first day of our program, Saturday, notice that the first segment of the day is breakfast. This is important. Eat breakfast as a family and eat breakfast immediately. To do so, you will want to choose light foods. Some suggestions are given in Chapter Five when we discuss the element of Diet/Nutrition. Family Fit suggests that breakfast contain food choices that are higher in carbohydrates. Why? Because as you will read in Chapter Five, Family Fit advocates a 40-40-20 balance for the entire day. (Most programs that propose similar food breakdowns talk about such divisions at each meal. Read the evidence presented in Chapter Five on why it is more effective to employ this breakdown over the course of a day.) That means 40 percent of your food choices should come from proteins, 40 percent from carbohydrates, and 20 percent from fat.

Carbohydrates provide energy. Concentrating carbohydrate consumption to the morning meal gives an energy boost. In addition to this needed fuel to start the day, this higher carbohydrate consumption in the morning addresses the concern of some other programs that advocate low carbohydrate consumption. It is true that if a person adheres to a super-high-carbohydrate diet with low protein and low fat, the carbohydrates your body doesn't use will put on weight. Furthermore, high carbohydrate foods are also generally high calorie foods, which supports the view that a diet concentrating on carbohydrates is not the answer to effective weight loss. In Family Fit, emphasizing that 40 percent of daily carbohydrates be eaten early in the day has the added benefit of using those carbohydrates up throughout the day both from daily body functions and in the Fitness Activity element of the Family Fit Program. These carbohydrates provide the energy needed to maintain your enthusiasm for the program.

Let's move to the next segment on the Day Planner. It is important to let that breakfast digest. To do this, the next segment of the day allows for relaxation, light morning chores such as taking care of the family pets, light house chores, or planning out the day. Any or all of these activities can be done together or individually depending on the nature of that activity and the needs of the family.

Remember, in Family Fit the clock is yours, not ours. You and your family set the exact times for these segments.

After this morning chore segment is complete, it is time for the family to participate in a fitness activity together. On this first Saturday, like all Saturdays in the program, your family activity should be longer. This means that this is a good day for a long hike in the park, a long bike ride, a family game outdoors, or a drive to get to a special place for a family activity that may require more time. The aim here is to place on Saturday or Sunday those fitness activities that would feel pinched on a more time-crunched weekday. In Chapter Seven suggestions and methods will be discussed for these family activities.

Moving forward on the Day Planner, when the family activity is finished, save time for rest, possibly other light individual chores, and other needs. The next family segment is lunch. This lunch should concentrate slightly more on proteins while continuing to keep carbohydrates high. This balance emphasizes recovery from the activity. Proteins are needed to restock energy and restore muscle exerted in the activity. The carbohydrates are needed to refuel, prepare for the rest of the day, and replenish the energy reserves.

Your family has eaten two meals together, done some chores (yes, children can and will do chores; see Chapter Nine for how this occurs), and participated together in a fitness activity (read in Chapter Seven why we are not emphasizing the word *exercise*), and you still have a day to enjoy. There are many options open for the rest of the day. If Saturday is not a workday for the adults in the family, now is the time to participate in your own projects, hobbies, and other household chores—in short, the all-American Saturday. Even if Saturday is a workday, there is no clock on the daily segments, so you go to work when scheduled. If you don't choose any of these options, how about just spending the rest of the day relaxing with your family? It is not sinful to participate in some sedentary activities, and now can be the time to do it. Play video games, watch TV, or go on the computer. So what? You have already been physically active.

In the next segment, family dinner, the family comes back together to eat. At this meal the 40-40-20 balance is stressed. Chapter Five will provide ideas on how to change old eating habits to fit this balance.

Modifications Are Okay

There are a few important considerations to mention right here. Families using Family Fit must adapt to the spontaneity in the lives of young family members. Someday every family in America will be following this program (we wish), but until then, young people will visit friends, attend birthday parties, and participate in other events that will keep them away from family meals and the Family Fit Program. But guess what? That's okay here. With some flexibility and accommodation, the majority of the Day Planner segments can be enjoyed. So a teen eats lunch on his or her own. Just remind him or her of what the parameters are in Family Fit. The same thinking applies to dinner. And here's the important ingredient. When teens do come home, ask them how they handled eating somewhere else and give them feedback.

Let's listen to a dad checking in with a typical teenager. "Hey, Peggy, what did you eat at the Flemmings'?"

Peggy answers, smiling, "Mrs. Flemming made one of those Hungry Man frozen dinners, and I didn't know what was in it. So I passed on that. They did set out a fresh salad and put bottles of salad dressing on the table. None of them were low fat or low cal, so I just ate the salad dry. They had enough stuff in it so it wasn't bad."

"Good job, I'm proud of you!" Dad says.

By the way, this checking in has a marvelous side effect—getting you very involved in your teens' lives. They will get used to you being involved with their activities.

Another consideration to mention here is the special event that arises for the entire family. If a special event is scheduled in the middle of a weekend day, just move the Family Fit segments around it. No problem.

An example of this type of special event is sporting events that school-age children participate in at school, at the YMCA, or at the community center. The flexibility of the Family Fit Program allows such events to be incorporated into the program. While the entire family attends these sporting events (something highly recommended to maintain family togetherness), the other members of the family can meet their activity needs. Many athletic events allow plenty of time and freedom for other family members to be active.

Little League for All

Pete, his wife, Maria, and their daughter, Christina, wouldn't think of missing one of Tony's Little League baseball games. These games were two hours long, and his team played thirty-six games over the summer. When Tony first started Little League, Pete and Maria were taken aback by the time commitment. After all, how would they get their own workouts in with so much time tied up in baseball? Pete came up with a brilliant solution. He suggested that Maria, Christina, and he dress in workout clothes when they attended Tony's games. By doing so, they could jog around the park during the game. They could meet their activity needs for that day and still support Tony in his sport. Now, at each game, Pete, Maria, and Christina watch as Tony and his teammates get ready for the game, then they all wait for a part of the game during which they feel comfortable taking thirty minutes to jog around the park. After their run, they stretch back by the diamond where Tony's team is playing, and they miss very little of the game. In fact, the park where most of the games are played is designed in such a way that the baseball field is always in view as the family jogs. They do not miss a single play of the game. And watching the game is a great way to break any monotony that a run may present. They all find that these runs seem to be the quickest and most enjoyable.

For Tony, a wonderful side benefit of this family activity is that he sees his family as an active, energetic group. Tony gets the message that his family values fitness and activity.

Almost any organized sport allows an opportunity for a family to meet their fitness/activity needs in the same manner. It may require you to be less inhibited about doing an activity in front of other spectators, but you will find that this is less of a concern than you would imagine. In fact, it's a wonderful example to set for the other families in attendance. In the case of Maria, Pete, and Christina, once they started jogging during the baseball games, they saw other families doing similar activities. Many spectators brought bikes and rode during the game, some brought baseball gloves of their own and played catch with each other, and other families could be seen kicking a soccer ball back and forth. The sidelines were abuzz with energy, and cheering for the team even increased as the spectators' activity levels increased.

The final segment of our first day is evening activities. The family has just finished dinner, and there is still an entire evening to be used as they please—together or separate, visiting friends, going to a movie, doing homework or office work, whatever. People complain that they don't have enough time for family and for exercise (pardon that word). You can see by this program that it can be done.

The second day of the Family Fit Program, Sunday, follows the first very closely. Breakfast is essentially the same, but a wonderful tradition that many families follow is the special homemade Sunday breakfast. Starting the Family Fit Program would be a great opportunity to rekindle this tradition in your family. If you are blending in family members from older generations, restarting this tradition on a Sunday morning is a great chance to welcome them into participating in your family's program.

The Sunday family fitness activity may repeat Saturday's longer fitness activity if everyone is in agreement. This is also a great opportunity to try something completely different.

After the family activity, you have the opportunity to copy another old family tradition—make Sunday lunch a brunch and turn it into the biggest meal of the day. If you do this, note the Day Planner suggests a light Sunday dinner. The remainder of Sunday follows the same Day Planner segments as Saturday.

Adding Work and School to the Equation

Now we come to the day that requires accommodation of work and school somewhere in the family's day—the infamous Monday. As previously discussed, Monday can be your family's day off from activity. What hasn't been mentioned yet is that if you are not making Monday your off day (which is highly suggested), then make sure you are making some other day during the week your day off. Try not to make Saturday or Sunday your off day because they traditionally offer that better time opportunity. Pick the day that will take the most pressure off your family. This will ensure that the program remains fun for everyone and never a burden.

Let's call Monday through Friday the midweek days. Breakfast during the midweek follows the same plan each day. Again, as during Saturday and Sunday, eat something immediately. Make these midweek breakfasts quick and easy but not boring. See Chapter Five for suggestions. The next daily segment replaces the segment in Saturday and Sunday in which light morning chores were done. During the midweek this segment comprises organizing and preparing for the day. During this time pack the school and work lunches, make sure the school bags and briefcases are organized, plan out the day, and look over your work schedule. Don't rush through these activities; remember this is also time for your breakfast to settle before your physical activity.

During the midweek, the family activity you choose should take into account the amount of time you have available. Don't plan something that will place you or other family members in a time crunch. Make it short but vigorous. See Chapter Seven for some suggestions.

Midweek lunch is also different. Family members basically have two choices during the midweek for lunch—make a lunch to take to work or school, or buy a lunch outside of the home. Family Fit advocates taking the lunch for obvious reasons. You can control what is in it, and you can make it tastier than a purchased lunch. But if the whole family or a single family member does opt to purchase lunch, then do the same type of advising that was advocated on the weekend when someone misses a meal. Remind them to eat healthy. Don't nag; just give a friendly reminder. Then when you are all together, either at dinnertime or at the end of the day, ask how they handled lunch. When you ask about this, do so with enthusiastic language and gestures. Don't let this checking in become a source of conflict. Compliment the family members on the choices they made and share with them how you handled your lunch.

The remainder of the day follows the pattern established on the first two days of the program. Family dinner is then followed by evening time. During the midweek, evening time will often be filled with homework, home-office work, chores, or entertainment.

A Family Day Planner that places the family activity later in the day is also provided. Note that meals have been adjusted to coordinate with this activity schedule. Do not eat heavy and still have a family activity coming up in your schedule. Family members will feel lethargic as a result and will lose motivation for the activity.

Family Day Planner (Week One)

	Saturday	Sunday	Monday
Breakfast	Eat immediately. Have foods that are higher in carbs. See chapter 5.	Eat immediately. Maybe a homemade treat that is higher in carbs? See chapter 5.	Eat immediately. Prepare quick foods higher in carbs. See chapter 5.
Morning	Plan day. Do house chores. Pet care?	Plan day. Do house chores. Pet care?	Pack lunch. Pack school bag/work materials.
Family Activity*	Activity should be longer in duration. Bike ride? Walk? Run? Hike? Swim?	Activity should be longer in duration. May repeat Saturday's activity if all agree. Or, try something new.	Take the day off? Some families may not want to take Monday off to keep motivation high, so go light.
Lunch	Meal should be higher in proteins.	Maybe brunch today? Main meal? Higher in proteins.	Eat separate lunch. See chapter 5.
Midday	Work on projects. Go shopping. Attend events. Visit friends.	Attend church or events. Relax. Entertain.	Work or school.
Dinner	Meal of 40-40-20 balance.	Light meal of 40-40-20 balance.	See chapter 5.
Evening	Have individual or family time. Do chores. Visit friends. Entertain.	Have individual or family time. Do chores. Visit friends. Entertain.	Do homework or chores.

Tuesday	Wednesday	Thursday	Friday
Eat immediately. Prepare quick foods higher in carbs. See chapter 5.	Eat immediately. Prepare quick foods higher in carbs. See chapter 5.	Eat immediately. Prepare quick foods higher in carbs. See chapter 5.	Eat immediately. Prepare quick foods higher in carbs. See chapter 5.
Pack lunch. Pack school bag/ work materials.	Pack lunch. Pack school bag/ work materials.	Pack lunch. Pack school bag/ work materials.	Pack lunch. Pack school bag/ work materials.
Vigorous and shorter duration. See chapter 7.	Vigorous and shorter duration. See chapter 7.	Vigorous and shorter duration. See chapter 7.	Vigorous and shorter duration. See chapter 7.
Eat separate lunch. See chapter 5.	Eat separate lunch. See chapter 5.	Eat separate lunch. See chapter 5.	Eat separate lunch. See chapter 5.
Work or school.	Work or school.	Work or school.	Work or school.
See chapter 5.	See chapter 5.	See chapter 5.	See chapter 5.
Do homework or chores.	Do homework or chores.	Do homework or chores.	Do homework or chores.

* The family activity can be placed in the evening; some families may find this more manageable. See the following page for a planner illustrating how to do this.

Family Day Planner (With Family Activity Placed Later in the Day)

	Saturday	Sunday	Monday*
Breakfast	Eat immediately. Have foods that are higher in carbs. See chapter 5.	Eat immediately. Maybe a homemade treat that is higher in carbs? See chapter 5.	Eat immediately. Prepare quick foods higher in carbs. See chapter 5.
Morning	Plan day. Do house chores. Pet care?	Plan day. Do house chores. Pet care?	Pack lunch. Pack school bag/ work materials.
Lunch	Meal should be higher in proteins.	Maybe brunch today? Main meal? Higher in proteins.	Eat separate lunch. See chapter 5.
Midday	Work on projects. Go shopping. Attend events. Visit friends. Family activity could also occur here.	Attend church or events. Relax. Entertain. Family activity could also occur here.	Work or school.
Family Activity	Activity should be longer in duration. Bike ride? Walk? Run? Hike? Swim?	Activity should be longer in duration. May repeat Saturday's activity if all agree. Or, try something new.	Take the day off? Some families may not want to take Monday off to keep motivation high, so go light.
Dinner	Eat a light family dinner.	Eat a light family dinner.	See chapter 5.
Evening	Have individual or family time. Do chores. Visit friends. Entertain.	Have individual or family time. Do chores. Visit friends. Entertain.	Do homework or chores.

Tuesday	Wednesday	Thursday	Friday
Eat immediately. Prepare quick foods higher in carbs. See chapter 5.	Eat immediately. Prepare quick foods higher in carbs. See chapter 5.	Eat immediately. Prepare quick foods higher in carbs. See chapter 5.	Eat immediately. Prepare quick foods higher in carbs. See chapter 5.
Pack lunch. Pack school bag/ work materials.	Pack lunch. Pack school bag/ work materials.	Pack lunch. Pack school bag/ work materials.	Pack lunch. Pack school bag/ work materials.
Eat separate lunch. See chapter 5.	Eat separate lunch. See chapter 5.	Eat separate lunch. See chapter 5.	Eat separate lunch. See chapter 5.
Work or school.	Work or school.	Work or school.	Work or school.
Vigorous and shorter duration. See chapter 7.	Vigorous and shorter duration. See chapter 7.	Vigorous and shorter duration. See chapter 7.	Vigorous and shorter duration. See chapter 7.
See chapter 5.	See chapter 5.	See chapter 5.	See chapter 5.
Do homework or chores.	Do homework or chores.	Do homework or chores.	Do homework or chores.

* Day off from activity?

On the following pages you will find Family Day Planners for weeks two and three of the Family Fit Program. The segments of Family Fit in weeks two and three are exactly the same as in week one. What changes in weeks two and three is the intensity of the family activities. Family members' bodies will quickly start to adapt to being active. In the second week of the program it is important to turn up the intensity a notch. Then in week three family members do the same. Turn the intensity up even further in the third week. By the third week of this program each family member should be active at a level that burns calories consistently. That means at least thirty minutes of aerobic activity six days a week. The Day Planner segments stay the same throughout the program. The eating habits of your family also stay consistent from the first day forward.

A word of caution as you look over all these Family Day Planners. Whenever a day is broken down and all the things we do in any given day are listed as was done here, it seems so ominous. Right now readers may be thinking, "Wow, I have to do all of this in a day for Family Fit?" "Oh, my God!" "How do I fit all of this in?" Guess what? Much of what is listed here is exactly what a typical family is doing in a day already without thinking about it.

> ***The Family Day Planners may look like a lot to do, but they actually just list everything we were doing in a typical day before starting Family Fit!***

Let's face it, in the typical household after breakfast and before going off and doing something, the pets may need to be walked and fed, the garbage may need to go out, and a load of laundry may have to be placed in the washing machine. You are doing these chores without thinking about them. The Family Day Planner calls attention to those needs that are part of the normal routine of family life. Incorporating the normal routine in this manner prevents the mistake of other programs, which don't address these normal needs and expect a family to follow a new lifestyle change as if that's all they have to do during the day. By putting normal family life right in the program, it extinguishes the common excuse of, "I don't have time for Family Fit." It's plain to see that there is plenty of time for Family Fit.

Family Day Planner (Week Two)

	Saturday	Sunday	Monday
Breakfast	Eat immediately. Have foods that are higher in carbs. See chapter 5.	Eat immediately. Maybe a homemade treat that is higher in carbs? See chapter 5.	Eat immediately. Prepare quick foods higher in carbs. See chapter 5.
Morning	Plan day. Do house chores. Pet care?	Plan day. Do house chores. Pet care?	Pack lunch. Pack school bag/work materials.
Family Activity* (Increase intensity of activity from last week. This is the only change from week to week.)	Activity should be longer in duration. Bike ride? Walk? Run? Hike? Swim?	Activity should be longer in duration. May repeat Saturday's activity if all agree. Or, try something new.	Take the day off? Some families may not want to take Monday off to keep motivation high, so go light.
Lunch	Meal should be higher in proteins.	Maybe brunch today? Main meal? Higher in proteins.	Eat separate lunch. See chapter 5.
Midday	Work on projects. Go shopping. Attend events. Visit friends.	Attend church or events. Relax. Entertain.	Work or school.
Dinner	Meal of 40-40-20 balance.	Light meal of 40-40-20 balance.	See chapter 5.
Evening	Have individual or family time. Do chores. Visit friends. Entertain.	Have individual or family time. Do chores. Visit friends. Entertain.	Do homework or chores.

Tuesday	Wednesday	Thursday	Friday
Eat immediately. Prepare quick foods higher in carbs. See chapter 5.	Eat immediately. Prepare quick foods higher in carbs. See chapter 5.	Eat immediately. Prepare quick foods higher in carbs. See chapter 5.	Eat immediately. Prepare quick foods higher in carbs. See chapter 5.
Pack lunch. Pack school bag/ work materials.	Pack lunch. Pack school bag/ work materials.	Pack lunch. Pack school bag/ work materials.	Pack lunch. Pack school bag/ work materials.
Vigorous and shorter duration than activity during weekend. See chapter 7.	Vigorous and shorter duration than activity during weekend. See chapter 7.	Vigorous and shorter duration than activity during weekend. See chapter 7.	Vigorous and shorter duration than activity during weekend. See chapter 7.
Eat separate lunch. See chapter 5.	Eat separate lunch. See chapter 5.	Eat separate lunch. See chapter 5.	Eat separate lunch. See chapter 5.
Work or school.	Work or school.	Work or school.	Work or school.
See chapter 5.	See chapter 5.	See chapter 5.	See chapter 5.
Do homework or chores.	Do homework or chores.	Do homework or chores.	Do homework or chores.

* The family activity can be placed in the evening; some families may find this more manageable. Adjust meals to accommodate.

Family Day Planner (Week Three)

	Saturday	Sunday	Monday
Breakfast	Eat immediately. Have foods that are higher in carbs. See chapter 5.	Eat immediately. Maybe a home-made treat that is higher in carbs? See chapter 5.	Eat immediately. Prepare quick foods higher in carbs. See chapter 5.
Morning	Plan day. Do house chores. Pet care?	Plan day. Do house chores. Pet care?	Pack lunch. Pack school bag/ work materials.
Family Activity* (Add a minimum of 30 minutes of activity in each fitness activity segment. Increase intensity of activity from last week.)	Activity should be longer in duration. Bike ride? Walk? Run? Hike? Swim?	Activity should be longer in duration. May repeat Saturday's activity if all agree. Or, try something new.	Take the day off? Some families may not want to take Monday off to keep motivation high, so go light.
Lunch	Meal should be higher in proteins.	Maybe brunch today? Main meal? Higher in proteins.	Eat separate lunch. See chapter 5.
Midday	Work on projects. Go shopping. Attend events. Visit friends.	Attend church or events. Relax. Entertain.	Work or school.
Dinner	Meal of 40-40-20 balance.	Light meal of 40-40-20 balance.	See chapter 5.
Evening	Have individual or family time. Do chores. Visit friends. Entertain.	Have individual or family time. Do chores. Visit friends. Entertain.	Do homework or chores.

Tuesday	Wednesday	Thursday	Friday
Eat immediately. Prepare quick foods higher in carbs. See chapter 5.	Eat immediately. Prepare quick foods higher in carbs. See chapter 5.	Eat immediately. Prepare quick foods higher in carbs. See chapter 5.	Eat immediately. Prepare quick foods higher in carbs. See chapter 5.
Pack lunch. Pack school bag/ work materials.	Pack lunch. Pack school bag/ work materials.	Pack lunch. Pack school bag/ work materials.	Pack lunch. Pack school bag/ work materials.
Vigorous and shorter duration than activity during weekend. See chapter 7.	Vigorous and shorter duration than activity during weekend. See chapter 7.	Vigorous and shorter duration than activity during weekend. See chapter 7.	Vigorous and shorter duration than activity during weekend. See chapter 7.
Eat separate lunch. See chapter 5.	Eat separate lunch. See chapter 5.	Eat separate lunch. See chapter 5.	Eat separate lunch. See chapter 5.
Work or school.	Work or school.	Work or school.	Work or school.
See chapter 5.	See chapter 5.	See chapter 5.	See chapter 5.
Do homework or chores.	Do homework or chores.	Do homework or chores.	Do homework or chores.

* The family activity can be placed in the evening; some families may find this more manageable. Adjust meals to accommodate.

Family Day Planner (Worksheet)

	Saturday	Sunday	Monday
Breakfast			
Morning			
Family Activity			
Lunch			
Midday			
Dinner			
Evening			

Tuesday	Wednesday	Thursday	Friday

To put Family Fit into perspective, let's take a look at how one family accomplishes the Family Day Planner. Below is an example of just the midweek portion of the Family Day Planner for the Hughes family.

	Monday	**Tuesday**	**Wednesday**	**Thursday**	**Friday**
6:30 a.m.	Breakfast.	Breakfast.	Breakfast.	Breakfast.	Breakfast.
6:45 a.m.	Organize/ prepare day.	Organize/ prepare day.	Organize/ prepare day.	Organize/ prepare day.	Organize/ prepare day.
7:00 a.m.	Family activity: off-day. Showers.	Family activity: aerobics with video (20 min.). Showers.	Family activity: aerobics with video (20 min.). Showers.	Family activity: aerobics with video (20 min.). Showers.	Family activity: aerobics with video (20 min.). Showers.
7:50 a.m.	Leave for work/ school.	Leave for work/ school.	Leave for work/ school.	Leave for work/ school.	Leave for work/ school.
12:00 p.m.	Lunch.	Lunch.	Lunch.	Lunch.	Lunch.
12:30 p.m.	Work/ school.	Work/ school.	Work/ school.	Work/ school.	Work/ school.
6:00 p.m.	Family dinner.	Family dinner.	Family dinner.	Family dinner.	Family dinner.
7:00 p.m.	Evening hours: homework or chores.	Evening hours: homework or chores.	Evening hours: homework or chores.	Evening hours: homework or chores.	Evening hours: homework or chores.
10:00 p.m.	Bedtime.	Bedtime.	Bedtime.	Bedtime.	Bedtime.

This is the overview of the Family Fit Program—three weeks of family activity, new eating habits, and motivation to change. Within these three weeks your family will see success by losing weight, toning their bodies, and having more cohesion as a family. These three weeks should be repeated over and over and used as a template for the remainder of your family life.

THINGS TO REMEMBER:
- Just remember threes:
  Three Pillars—Three Fortifiers—Three Weeks.
- Fill out your Family Day Planner.
- Eat 40-40-20 over the whole day, not at each meal.
- The Diet/Nutrition pillar is fortified by New Habits, Cleanup, and Forward Thinking.
- The Activity pillar is fortified by Individual Goals, Family Goals, and Generational Goals.
- The Motivation pillar is fortified by Your Surroundings, Self-Motivation, and Person-to-Person Motivation.

PART III

THREE WEEKS AND THREE WAYS TO SUCCESS: THE FAMILY FIT PROGRAM

CHAPTER FIVE

The First Way—The Diet and Nutrition Pillar

Diet and Nutrition constitutes the first pillar of the Family Fit Program. Clearly, what we put into our bodies is the foundation of how we end the painful cycle of obesity. It is fitting that we start the description of our program with this important topic. Crafting a new eating lifestyle brings new energy and life into the family that will be important for putting in place the two other pillars of the Family Fit Program.

New Habits

The vast majority of people who have been caught in the generational cycle of obesity have tried many diets in their lifetimes. They are quite knowledgeable about foods, calories, and fat content. This chapter will make some assumptions based on this knowledge. This chapter will also present new information based on the latest research findings. The foundation of our approach to eating is simple. Eat healthy, increase your level of physical activity, and *enjoy eating*, and you will lose weight. Enjoyment cannot be stressed enough. Traditional diets fail because they are restrictive, and people have to sacrifice enjoyment and comfort to participate in them. Eating should be fun and pleasurable. Any program that doesn't recognize this will fail. In Family Fit eating, you do not have to restrict yourself or sacrifice. All you have to do is think. Do you enjoy a certain food or taste? This chapter will show you how you can continue enjoying it but make it healthier for you and your family with a little thought.

A way that eating has not been fun for dieters recently has resulted from the confusion surrounding the proper balance between carbohydrates, proteins, and fats. One diet advocates all protein, another all carbohydrates, and still another shockingly says to eat all the fat you want. Let's end this confusion right here. The Family Fit approach knows that healthy eating results from a balance in your food intake of 40 percent proteins, 40 percent carbohydrates, and no more than 20 percent fats. These figures are based on the medical evidence of how your body works most efficiently, so let's not get caught up in the debate of which should be higher, protein or carbohydrates. If you eat equal amounts of both and keep your fat intake low (around 20 percent of everything you eat), reduce the amount of calories you take in each day, and increase your physical activity, you will not only lose weight but also maintain a lifelong healthy eating plan.

Balancing Act

Carbohydrates and proteins have been grabbing the headlines lately in diet programs, but our knowledge and use of fat needs to be better understood. Physiologically, approximately 4 to 5 percent of your daily calories *must* come from fat in order to provide the body with essential nutrients. Specifically, fatty acids come from our intake of fat. Fatty acids are necessary for the healthy functioning of your body because they are one of the body's building blocks. Fat in your diet is essential to absorb and use many vitamins and minerals, including vitamins A, D, E, and K. These fat-soluble vitamins help with vision, the immune system, and the reproductive system. Fat is a fundamental component of myelin, the material that coats nerve cells. Fat adds to the flavor of foods. It is false to think that you don't need any fat in your diet. The problem begins when we eat too much fat and the wrong type of fat.

Dietary fat is divided into three types—saturated fats, unsaturated fats, and trans-unsaturated fats, or trans-fatty acids. Saturated fats and unsaturated fats are natural substances found in food products. Saturated fats are the enemies here. These fats have long been associated with heart disease and high cholesterol levels.

Unsaturated fats are friendlier to us. Unsaturated fats are further divided into polyunsaturated fats and monounsaturated fats. Monounsaturated fats are found in olives, peanuts, and avocados. Polyunsaturated fats are linoleic fat (also called omega-6, found in corn, soy, and other vegetables) and alpha-linoleic, or omega-3, fat. Omega-3 fat is the best of all the fats. It is found in flax and cold-water fishes. These unsaturated fats help raise the HDL cholesterol level. HDL cholesterol is good for our bodies because it helps keep arteries clean and the heart healthy. Omega-3 fat does this the best.

It is very important to note that just because unsaturated fats are better for us does not mean that we should eat all we want of them. In the past, people have been tricked into thinking that you can eat all you want of these good fats. People think this has given them permission to eat large quantities of low-fat or fat-free foods, which means large numbers of calories. They thought that by eating unsaturated fats they would automatically lose weight without worrying about the quantities of food they consumed. The truth is that saturated and unsaturated fats have basically the same amount of calories.

Avoid at All Costs

Trans-unsaturated fats are the result of a food production method that changes liquid unsaturated fats into solid foods or foods that have a thicker density. This process is used to make food better for cooking and spreading on things. The problem is, this process turns the liquid unsaturated fats into fats that resemble saturated fats. Digested, these trans-unsaturated fats are the equivalent of saturated fats and they should be avoided. You will find these trans-unsaturated fats in margarine, frozen meals, and deep-fried foods among others. Look carefully on food labels to discover the amounts of these three fats in the contents of the food you buy.

Cholesterol and Fat Intake

Researchers are discovering that if a person's daily fat consumption drops too low, even to 10 or 12 percent, that person's HDL (good) cholesterol levels will begin to drop, in addition to the other effects mentioned earlier. So, again, some fat is good, but be careful. Our guideline of 20 percent fat per day from your food is a safe, low level of fat consumption for all family members. In fact, we have been a bit manipulative in setting that figure at 20 percent. The American diet is so rich in fat that it is very hard to reach the goal of 20 percent without very restrictive eating. There are many foods, even in healthy diets, which have hidden fat content. The goal of 20 percent is a target to aim at, but if your family achieves a level of 25 percent, you will be well within a healthier lifestyle and will reduce your LDL (bad) cholesterol level by as much as 15 percent.

Putting these percentages into quantities is not that difficult. Determine how many calories you are going to consume in a day (this calculation is given later in the book), take that number and multiply it by 20 percent (.20). Take the resulting number and divide that by nine, which is the number of calories in each gram of fat. The final number will give you the amount, in grams, of fat you should be eating each day.

As an example, if you have determined that your goal is to eat 2,000 calories a day, multiply 2,000 by .20. This equals 400. Now take 400 and divide by 9. The result is 44 grams of fat per day.

FAT GRAM CALCULATOR

Number of calories per day × .20 = A

A ÷ 9 = Number of fat grams allowed each day

The needs of children do not differ in terms of the total amount of fat they should be eating each day. The exception here is that children under the age of two should not be concerned about restricting fats at all. Children older than two should follow the same daily percentage of fat intake as adults.

Fatty foods (those with high saturated fat content) are also typically high-calorie foods. Because of this high correlation between high fat and high calorie, eliminating fatty foods is an important goal of the Family Fit plan for a healthier family lifestyle. To help eliminate as many fatty foods as possible, the following pages contain a list of ways to reduce fat in your diet.

WAYS TO REDUCE FAT IN YOUR FAMILY DIET

1. Cut in half the amount of butter, margarine, oil, or shortening you use in all recipes. You will not lose flavor by doing so. Try using one of the newly developed substitute products that have no fat. Their taste and consistency has come a long way in just the last few years. They will work in recipes.

2. Buy lean meats. In beef the leanest cuts are round and sirloin. In pork the leanest cuts are loin and tenderloin. In lamb the leanest is the shank. In veal most cuts are lean, although the rib sections can be fatty. For all meats shop for the highest grade available.

3. Don't cook pasta, rice, or noodles with butter, oil, or shortening even though the package says to do so. You will not lose any taste. Don't get caught by the fallacy that adding these things will keep the pasta from sticking. The only things you can do to avoid sticking in pasta and noodles are to serve them right out of the boiling water or use a rinse of hot water. For rice use a rice cooker.

4. In chicken and turkey buy the white meat.

5. Remove the skin from all poultry before cooking.

6. Say good-bye to hot dogs, except fat-free hot dogs.

7. Buy 1 percent or 2 percent milk. There is no doubt that the taste is different, but you are saving your family loads of fat each day. Use this type of milk for all your cooking as well. Milk is a great, wholesome food when used this way.

8. Cheese is a word to take right out of your family's food encyclopedia. Fat-free cheeses are an adequate substitute, but to make them fat-free, they typically have a high water content and can't be used in some recipes or don't melt the same as regular cheese does. Experiment here and be patient. You will probably see better versions of fat-free or low-fat cheeses soon.

9. Avoid traditional brands of white bread. Besides the fact that processed white flour is not the best choice for your body, traditional white bread adds calories and fat to the diet. Wheat bread, English muffins, bagels, stone-ground breads, and seven-grain breads are better choices.

10. Speaking of breads, have you ever eaten bread without butter or a spread? Voila! You will be surprised that bread tastes great without anything topping it. This is particularly true if it is a homemade bread. If you must top bread, use fruit "butters," which are typically low fat. For breakfast try your toast with low-fat or fat-free jam. It tastes great!

11. Like bread, when was the last time you tasted a potato? That is, just a potato—no butter, sour cream, chives, or bacon bits. Potatoes have gotten a very bad reputation, in part because of all the junk we have automatically piled on them for generations. In doing so, we have lost the taste of a potato. Try it—bake a potato and eat it plain. A bit of salt and pepper will also add great taste.

12. Mayonnaise, like cheese, is a word to rip right out of the family food encyclopedia. Fat-free mayonnaise has come light years in taste in the last several years.

13. Throw out that jar of traditional peanut butter. Buy reduced-fat peanut butter, but watch the brand. Some brands have higher calories than others.

14. No more cream in coffee. Use powdered fat-free substitutes, which have come a long, long way in flavor, or use your 2 percent milk. Better yet, really taste the coffee and drink it black.

15. If a recipe calls for cream, you can generally substitute it with evaporated skim milk.

16. Desserts? Don't even think about them. If your family has a sweet tooth that has been trained to expect satisfaction after a meal, fresh fruit is a great substitute.

17. You can make a great salad dressing by tossing the salad with wine vinegar and then sprinkling it with Equal. This little trick has zero calories and no fat. And surprise! It tastes good. An even simpler salad dressing with no calories and no fat is made with balsamic vinegar. Simply sprinkle balsamic vinegar over your salad greens and you have a tasty, easy dressing.

18. Cream sauces are deadly. Alfredo sauce is the biggest culprit. A small serving of fettuccine with Alfredo sauce has approximately 100 grams of fat—almost three days' worth. Head for tomato-based sauces, but watch that they are not made with cream.

19. Be careful of yogurt. Regular yogurt is high in fat and calories. Eat low-fat or fat-free yogurt, but even here watch the brand. Some brands of low-fat yogurt are high in calories, especially for the amount you would need to consume to fill you up.

20. When dining out, don't order anything fried.

21. When dining out, be careful of taco salads. They often come served in that festive deep-fried taco shell. That taco shell just wiped out two days' worth of watching your fat intake.

22. If you like Chinese take-out, only order those dishes that are steamed (usually a great choice), boiled, or stir-fried. But tell them to stir-fry your order in lemongrass water or anything but oil.

23. You can still have pizza, but start by not having sausage on it. Try Canadian bacon instead, and if they don't have a low-fat cheese to use as a substitute, then tell them no cheese. You will be surprised how good pizza tastes with no cheese. Zero in on the menu at pizza places for new, California-style pizzas that are not made with the traditional fatty ingredients. Many restaurants across the country are serving these.

24. At the movies, do not eat the popcorn unless you see air-popped versions without added butter.

25. When dining out, many people are fooled into thinking that they are being healthful by concentrating on salads at restaurants. The danger here is that salads at many restaurants are just as caloric and fatty as many other choices on the menu. This is primarily because restaurant salad dressings are typically horrible for you. They are high in calories and fat because they are oil or mayonnaise based. Some oils, such as canola, sunflower, safflower, corn soy, and olive oils, are better in moderation. Most restaurants opt for the cheaper hydrogenated oils that are higher in fat and calories. Restaurants also love to add cheese, bacon bits, fried croutons, luncheon meats, or other ingredients that just boost the fat and calorie content through the roof.

As we discuss new habits about food, our first target has been fatty foods not only because their name is synonymous with obesity, but also because it has long been recognized by medical science that our diet is much too rich in fats. Notice that any discussion of fats cannot help but bring up calories. That's because fat contains twice as many calories as carbohydrates and proteins. New habits in eating must concentrate on calories and total food intake. In the Family Fit plan it is important for family members to be aware of their total number of daily calories. Calories can be viewed as fuel cells or energy capsules. They are burned to fuel the body. Anything over the amount needed to fuel the body will be stored for possible later use. If not used, they are stored as body fat.

Calculating the number of calories you should be consuming can be done with a simple formula. For an adult who is sedentary, take your present weight and multiply it by 14. For moderately active adults (those who exercise aerobically three to four times per week), multiply your weight by 17. And for active adults (those who aerobically exercise five to seven times per week), multiply your weight by 20. This is the total number of calories your body requires to keep basic bodily functions going. This is called the basal metabolic rate (BMR).

For example, for a female adult who weighs 130 pounds and is moderately active, the formula is 130 times 17; this equals 2,210 calories. For an adult male of 200 pounds who is sedentary, the formula is 200 times 14. This equals a total of 2,800 calories per day.

CALORIE CALCULATOR

weight	x	14 (sedentary) 17 (moderately active) 20 (active)	=	number of calories per day

Children's and teens' basic calorie needs are slightly different than adults. The Food and Nutrition Board of the National Academy of Sciences estimates the recommended calorie intakes for young people as listed in the following chart.

RECOMMENDED CALORIE INTAKE FOR YOUNG PEOPLE

Age	Calories per Pound	Average per Day
0 – 6 months	49	650
6 months – 1 year	45	850
1 – 3 years	46	1,300
4 – 6 years	41	1,800
7 – 10 years	32	2,000
11 – 14 years (boys)	25	2,500
15 – 18 years (boys)	20	3,000
11 – 14 years (girls)	21	2,200
15 – 18 years (girls)	18	2,200

In both adults and children, the daily calorie needs given in the above charts provide a good estimate of the amount of calories the body needs to maintain basic functions (BMR). If an individual consumes fewer calories than the body needs, then the body will go to the reserves stored as fat to make up the difference. Dipping into the reserves has always been the traditional goal of dieting. If you take in less than the basic number of calories needed for basic functions (BMR), you will lose weight. In the Family Fit Program our goal is the same. If each family member takes in fewer calories than expended daily, each family member will lose weight, tone the body, and stay healthy. Once family members reach their desired weight and body shape, then the goal is to maintain approximately the number of calories needed to sustain BMR and the new increased level of physical activity.

One of the fundamental ways that the Family Fit Program differs from other weight loss programs is we concern ourselves with eating over the entire day rather than concentrating on individual meals. The 40-40-20 balance advocated by the Family Fit Program looks at 40-40-20 as a *daily* recommendation. In Chapter Four, the program overview, the Family Day Planner suggested that certain meals stress one food group over another for that meal. This means each meal would not follow 40-40-20, but would have a proportion suitable to the needs of that time of day. For example, breakfast should contain higher carbohydrates so that the energy needed for the day is loaded into the body and then burned off by the day's activities. That may make the food balance of breakfast something like 70 percent carbohydrates, 20 percent proteins, and 10 percent fats. Then, the Family Day Planner suggests that lunch (when the family activity is undertaken in the morning) emphasize proteins over carbohydrates and fats. Lunch may then result in a balance of 30 percent carbohydrates, 60 percent proteins, and 10 percent fats. The important consideration is that at the end of the day each family member is at 40-40-20. This takes the stress out of individual meals. Did you eat more carbohydrates at lunch than you intend to? Simply adjust the balance at dinner. Was breakfast higher in protein today than you would have liked? Make sure lunch emphasizes your carbohydrate intake. The day becomes a balance of food intake.

This perspective over the entire day also helps prevent failure through the "I've already blown it" excuse. This excuse is common to all addictions, and obesity is no exception. A person makes a mistake at one point in the day and then says, "Well, I've ruined this day, so I may as well do what I want for the rest of the day." They take this attitude and compound the mistake by eating unhealthy for the rest of the day, and usually this unhealthy eating is not just tiny indiscretions; we're talking about major pig-outs.

Another method of charting a healthy body is through the calculation of the body mass index (BMI). You can figure your BMI by taking your weight in pounds and multiplying it by 703. Divide the result by your height in inches. Divide this result by your height in inches again. Now you have your BMI. If your BMI is between 17 and 24, you're at a good weight. If your BMI is 25 or more, you are overweight. If your BMI is 30, you are obese.

BMI CALCULATOR

weight × 703 = A

A ÷ height (in inches) = B

B ÷ height (in inches) = BMI

BMI 17–24 = healthy weight
BMI 25–29 = overweight
BMI 30 and up = obese

The BMI is an excellent gauge of appropriate body weight. The BMI can be calculated for children, but the formula is different than that which is used for adults. Divide the child's weight (in pounds) by the squared sum of his or her height (in inches). Take that result and multiply it by the number 703. This will give you the child's BMI. Unlike the adult BMI, where increases signal a problem, a child's BMI should go up as she ages.

Do not use adult BMI standards as your measure for children!

Warning!
In order to include all family members in every phase of this program and because the Body Mass Index is an important measure of adult health, we provide this BMI calculation for children. Remember, a child's BMI should change as they grow, but sudden drastic changes could signal a problem.

CHILD'S BMI CALCULATOR

weight (in pounds) ÷ height (in inches)^2 × 703 = BMI

Cleanup
In Chapter Three, cleanup of the home and environment was discussed in a global way. Here we would like to discuss cleanup of foods that are offensive to the Family Fit Program. Cleanup is one of the three tools of Diet and Nutrition. Food cleanup is essential to success.

If an unhealthy food doesn't get into the home, then it cannot get into the mouth.

It is amazing how many families struggle with establishing a healthy lifestyle, and if you looked into their cupboards, you would find all kinds of fattening foods. On the next page is a chart that suggests foods that need to be swept from the house. Do this immediately with no excuses.

Certainly this chart does not cover all the foods that we need to sweep out of our homes. These are the most traditional mistakes. The fun of Family Fit is to play with foods. This takes us back to when families were creative with food, tried new things, and experimented with preparations. Unfortunately, in those days nutritional knowledge was primitive. But how families approached food and eating was more creative, artistic, and in general more fun. What you create today can be just as exciting as in yesteryear, and now it can be healthy too. Pull the family into this creative effort. Ask for their ideas and suggestions. Be creative with food. Don't be afraid to make mistakes. Mistakes can be part of the fun.

FOODS TO SWEEP FROM THE HOME

Food	Why
Butter	There are better ways to enhance foods and recipes.
Sodas	They contain empty calories and empty nutrition.
Peanut butter	It's much too fatty and caloric.
Whole milk	It's much too fatty and caloric.
Cream	There are lower-fat alternatives for flavoring your coffee.
Beef burgers	Red meat is too high in fat.
Beef chili	Red meat is too high in fat.
Candy bars	There are healthier ways to satisfy a sweet tooth.
Salad dressings	Be careful here! Salads lose their innocence because of dressings that are high in calories and fat.
Bread and rolls	There are healthier alternatives.
Desserts	Watch traditional desserts. Nothing wrong with this course at a meal; just do it more healthfully.
Boxed macaroni and cheese	Not healthy as is.
Fried chicken and other fried foods	They have added fat and calories.

Substitute

Try light butter, with no more than 3 percent saturated fat. Or try tasting foods without butter. Some low-fat and nonfat butter substitutes have higher saturated fat contents than light butter from traditional suppliers such as Land-O-Lakes.

Drink water (the best), diet sodas, or juices.

Try low-fat peanut butter, honey, or apple butter.

Try 1 percent, 2 percent, or fat-free milk (the taste is getting better).

Use nondairy powdered creamer, but read the label; light creams; or light or nonfat whipping cream—fun and healthy!

Substitute turkey or chicken burger, or if you must, use ¾ turkey and ¼ beef.

Use ground turkey instead of ground beef. Your sauce makes the dish, not the meat.

Slim-Fast Peanut Butter Crunch Bar—try it! It tastes just like a Butterfinger. And it's good for your family. But avoid the other flavors of their bars; some taste like chalk.

Nonfat dressings have come light years in taste. Try balsamic vinegar alone. Or mix nonfat mayonnaise with herbs such as chives, tarragon, or chili pepper, or else experiment. It's fun!

Homemade breads—wheat or seven-grain; nothing with white flour. Serve plain; there's no need for butter.

Fruit course; why eat some raspberry-flavored thing when you can enjoy the real thing? When was the last time your family tasted the real flavors of fruits instead of manufactured flavors?

Make your own; it's just as quick. Use light or nonfat cheeses, and be creative. Or make a fast alio olio: Take any style of pasta and lightly season with virgin olive oil, garlic, and your favorite herbs, such as oregano and basil.

Bake foods and use seasonings to create that taste you want. Do not buy any form of ready-made chicken at grocery stores or fast-food places unless you can read a nutritional label on fat and calorie content.

FOODS TO SWEEP FROM THE HOME

Food	Why
Mayonnaise	Traditional mayonnaise is very high in fat and calories.
Hot dogs	They have little nutritional value and are too high in fat and calories.
Alcoholic beverages	They're filled with empty calories.
Potato chips	A snack very high in fat and calories; there are better choices available.
Dip	Like salad dressings, be careful because these are often paired with healthy foods.
Mashed potatoes	When made traditionally, they're unhealthy.
French fries	When made traditionally, they're unhealthy.
Au gratin potatoes	When made traditionally, they're very unhealthy.
Sauces	These usually contain needless calories and fat.
Snack cakes	These have empty, needless calories. Don't give to kids as a treat!
Pizza	Often made carelessly, pizza can be a greasy, fat-laden calorie bomb.
Cheese	Whole-milk based cheeses are not right for the program.
Sour cream	It's too fatty and caloric.

Substitute

Use brown mustard to flavor sandwiches or one of hundreds of flavored mustards now sold everywhere. Make your sandwiches more interesting and no one will miss mayonnaise. Use low-fat and no-fat mayonnaise.

Turkey dogs. Oscar Meyer Fat-Free Hot Dogs actually taste good!

Wine in moderation. Mineral waters with lemon.

Try low-calorie baked chips or tortilla chips, but read the label.

Substitute salsas, preferably homemade. Try making or buying fruit salsas.

Use 2 percent milk or chicken broth (restaurants do) and no butter, or if you must, use light butter. Try mashed sweet potatoes; mash just the potatoes.

Only eat homemade baked "fries." Cut the potato strips bigger; baking will shrink them. Try baked sweet potatoes; they're sweeter and stay juicier.

Can still have these; just don't buy the boxed store version. Like macaroni and cheese, these are too fast and easy not to make yourself. Use sliced potatoes, 2 percent milk, a touch of olive oil for the baking dish, and fat-free cheeses.

Any sauce can be made healthier. Don't use pan drippings. Use only low-calorie, low-fat ingredients. You can reproduce any sauce, gravy, or topping.

Better snacks and lunch-box treats include sliced apples with low-fat peanut butter, flavored rice cakes (only buy healthy ones). Rice cakes can taste like popcorn, but some flavors are bland or tasteless.

Substitute Canadian bacon for Italian sausage. Try it without cheese. Make your own. Try California-style pizzas.

Use only low-fat, light cheeses. Or go without cheese.

Use low-fat yogurt or light or low-fat sour cream.

Food Should Be Fun!

One morning in the Dylan household, Eddie, age ten, received the task of fixing the family breakfast after days of begging for permission. The rest of the Dylans were a bit taken aback when they arrived at the table to discover that Eddie had made eggs with a dash of soy sauce. The combination seemed a bit unusual, and they all had a giggle over it. Nonetheless, they ate it and enjoyed it—much to the delight of Eddie. A few years later, one evening while they were watching the news on TV, a food critic was heaping effusive praise on a local restaurant because of its unique flair with food. One of the dishes that the critic just couldn't praise enough was a lunch entrée of eggs sprinkled with soy sauce. The Dylans all laughed and teased Eddie about what a trendsetter he was.

Is food fun if you rush home, take out a box from the freezer, rip it open, throw it in the microwave, blast it with intense radiation, take it out, dump the container into a serving bowl, line up your family to take a portion, and ingest it within three minutes? This picture just doesn't seem like fun.

Instead, when you arrive home let each family member take an item to prepare in her own style and flair. Someone makes the entrée, another family member the vegetable course, another the salad, another prepares the bread, another is in charge of garnishing every plate with some sliced raw vegetables, and yet another prepares a dessert.

As the meal comes together, the family will anticipate eating it. Maybe you will giggle a bit at the creations of a young family member, just like Eddie above with his soy eggs. And the result is that everyone will feel good about his own creation for this quick family meal. Teenage Sue beams as she brings to the table her entrée of pasta with garlic, olive oil, peas, and pearl onions. Billy, also a teen, feels like Emeril as he puts his colorful mini-chopped salad on each side dish. Mom can get a bit creative and add sliced raw almonds to the green beans she steamed. Little nine-year-old Becky circles everyone's plate with sliced carrots, making an edible colorful orange bouquet to surround the food. Everyone gets a slice of toasted seven-grain bread that Timmy, age seven, made in the toaster and smeared with a dab of honey. And for dessert, Dad prepares his famous Matterhorns, which are actually individual cups of coconut Jell-O with peaks of fat-free whipped cream (Dad is an engineer, this is as creative as he gets!). Can you imagine the smiles and the natural conversation that will ensue as the family sits down to eat this extravaganza? And it took about the same time as plopping that box in the microwave.

Life is too difficult to take away something that makes us all feel good. Bring back the enjoyment of food. Too many people today react to food as if they hate it. "Ugh…that's so much trouble to make." "God…I still have to make dinner when I get home. Can't somebody else cook?" With the fast-food mentality, we don't even look at our food anymore; it is just shoved in our mouths without thought. If food is so much drudgery and you hate playing with it so much, well…don't eat! No one is forcing food down your gullet. Let's stop this war against food in our families and let's begin to enjoy food. This is an important, healthy lifestyle message to give to young family members. Don't let them grow up with negative attitudes about food. These negative attitudes perpetuate the painful cycle of obesity in our families.

Water

One food mentioned on the preceding chart deserves special attention in our families—water. Water is often neglected in households. It has been consistently shown to be as good a thirst quencher as any sports drink or other beverage. We just do not drink enough water in our diet even though it is vital to our physical well-being. Make sure your family drinks plenty. The average healthy adult should drink the equivalent of about two quarts of water per day. For family members of all ages, the recommendation is one quart of water for each 1,000 calories of food consumed in the day.

All food and beverages contain water, but thinking that you will get your necessary amount of daily water from just eating or drinking beverages is false. The most beneficial effects of water are derived from drinking it unadulterated with no added sugar or flavoring.

Water's benefits are quite numerous. Water balances the electrolytes of the body. Electrolytes are minerals such as sodium, chloride, and potassium. These electrolytes help regulate body temperature and control blood pressure. Water is also essential for the transportation of water-soluble vitamins and nutrients such as proteins, minerals, and vitamins B and C. Water is a significant source of vital nutrients that are difficult to obtain from other sources. These are magnesium, cobalt, copper, and manganese.

Dehydration, a condition that arises when the body's cells are starving for water, can often be confused with hunger pains. A one percent drop in the body's fluid volume can noticeably reduce your body's ability to perform its vital functions. A 4 percent drop in body fluid volume reduces by one-third the body's ability to perform its vital functions. Keeping the body hydrated is essential and should be stressed in your family.

Special circumstances require special water needs. When exercising, the need for water is paramount. Water helps the muscles recover quickly from exercise and restores the body fluid volume lost through sweating. One should drink eight ounces of water for every half hour of exercise.

Pregnant women or women who are breast-feeding should add at least sixteen ounces of water to the two-quart daily recommendation for the average adult. Increased water consumption in pregnancy can help prevent the symptoms of morning sickness.

When reducing your calorie intake, such as when starting our Family Fit Program here, it is very important to increase water intake for a number of reasons. When we diet, more uric acid builds up in the bloodstream, which can cause kidney stones. Drinking water will flush out the uric acid, preventing stones. When dieting, water keeps your stomach full and prevents hunger. A glass of water fifteen minutes before each meal will help reduce overeating (Grandpa Mayer's Disease).

Other circumstances that require extra water intake are winter weather, as the indoor environment becomes drier; traveling, particularly in aircraft; and hot, humid weather, as we lose fluids through sweating.

Serve water with meals. As mentioned above, an old trick in the dieting field is to drink a full glass of water fifteen minutes before a meal to reduce the quantity of food you eat. In fact, many of these snake-oil-like diet pills instruct you to take them just like that; that is, with a full glass of water right before you eat. Well, guess what? Some of these magic pills are almost useless, and it's the water that is really helping you reduce your food intake. So save your money and use the magic appetite suppressor that's free—water.

Vitamin and Mineral Supplements

A debate that continually rages in nutrition circles is the question of vitamin supplements in our diets. Family Fit believes in vitamin supplements for several reasons. Most Americans do not get all their nutrients from the foods they eat. Even when changing old habits as we are outlining here in Family Fit, it is difficult to ensure that your body is getting the optimum vitamin and mineral requirements it needs to maximize health.

Some of the food substitutions you can make to cut calories and fat may take with them vitamins and minerals that the fatty, caloric food also contained. Often this is unavoidable. Instead of trading off these vitamins and minerals to save on calories and fat, take a vitamin supplement.

The final argument for vitamin and mineral supplements is that without all the necessary vitamins and minerals your body needs, you can actually gain weight. Your body is a magnificent machine. If it has a deficit, it will seek aggressively to fill that loss. Research shows that vitamin and mineral deficiencies can create cravings for foods. Often these cravings get translated into our brains as needs for unhealthy foods.

Scientists are now postulating that a pregnant woman's cravings may be explained by vitamin and mineral deficiencies. The pregnant body needs extra nutrients, which gets translated in ways not yet understood into cravings for particular foods. Ever known a woman who craved chocolate-covered bananas while pregnant? It's common because that indulgence contains a great deal of potassium. Ice cream cravings? This satisfies the need for extra calcium. How about the mom-to-be who becomes a fiend for red meat—the rarer the better? Rare red meat contains loads of iron. Iron forms hemoglobin, which carries oxygen to the bloodstream. Added iron is critical during pregnancy as the woman's blood supply is now being shared with the fetus.

Vitamin supplements are a good idea for the whole family. Buy vitamin and mineral supplements that come from natural sources, and use a daily multivitamin. Loading up on specific vitamins in addition to your family's healthier eating habits with Family Fit is not just overkill: Medical science is finding out that overloading on vitamins can lead to organ damage and other serious illnesses over time. One multivitamin from natural sources daily is easy and ensures that family members receive everything they need to stay healthy.

Forward Thinking

The third tool bolstering the family's Diet and Nutrition program is Forward Thinking. Forward thinking involves thinking ahead about eating situations. One of the many causes of our generational obesity has been the abundance of food we enjoy in modern life. Because food is plentiful, we have begun to take it for granted. This wasn't the case in our grandparents' generation. Not many years ago gathering, preparing, and eating food was something that took a great deal of planning and thought throughout the family's day. Food wasn't as available. Food couldn't be stored as efficiently. Varieties of food couldn't be obtained at certain times of the year. Methods of cooking foods took time, preparation, and planning. Food was a daily chore in the family. As a result, people thought ahead about their meals and their food. Today, this couldn't be further from the truth. So many family members spend no time at all thinking ahead about what they are going to eat, and because food is so plentiful when a mealtime arrives in their day, they just make impulsive, spontaneous decisions. This situation greatly contributes to poor food choices and obesity. Instead of food being thought out, it is incidental to the day's activities. Stopping this habit will help the family stop obesity.

The solution is to lead family members into thinking more about food and the choices they are going to make in the day. Make forward thinking a topic of family discussion. It gives the family something to talk about together. It provides a family focus. "Oh, Bill…you're going to that conference today. What will you do for lunch?" "Hey, Jesse, that field trip is tomorrow. Don't forget that at the museum all they have are those horrid hot dogs and hamburgers at that basement cafeteria. That place smells, too. Can you take a lunch with you? Why don't you find out today in school?"

In Chapter Four other forms of forward thinking were discussed, such as the family party and the special event. In that section, control and thinking ahead were discussed as remedies for the unhealthy choices you may be confronted with at such places. Family discussion is a great way to tease out the pitfalls of such events. Encourage your family to talk about these events and visualize how they will apply Family Fit prior to the occasion. It is a great exercise to use all the time. Forward thinking keeps your family right on track with your Family Fit Program.

More Diet/Nutrition Tips

Breakfast: Breakfast has been emphasized in Family Fit because of its great utility in fueling the body for the day. Skipping breakfast starts the day at a nutrition deficit that can lead right back into old, unhealthy habits. Without breakfast you decrease your energy base, you lose motivation, and cravings can start as your body tries to make up for these deficits.

To keep carbohydrates emphasized at breakfast this is a good time to eat breads, cereals, fruit, and juices. All of these selections are fast, high in carbohydrates, and filling. A banana, apple, and juice is an energy bomb for the body, and it is quick and easy in the morning rush.

Cereal is also quick and easy to prepare, but have you ever tried cereal without milk? Take a portion of your favorite healthy cereal and place it in a large cup. Pressed for time? While you are doing those light morning chores as outlined on the Family Day Planner, you can carry the cup around with you and shake out mouthfuls at your leisure. No more cereal sitting in soggy milk. It's not only a real time saver, but it's good nutrition as well. Kids will love it if you bring them their favorite cereal in their own cup when you wake them in the morning. They can start their breakfast right after you wake them up just like the Family Day Planner advises.

Another quick, easy, nutritious breakfast that can be eaten right out of a cup is a homemade smoothie. Throw two cups of frozen mixed berries, a banana, a cup of low-fat yogurt, one cup of your favorite juice, and some ice into the blender. Flip the switch and in minutes you have breakfast for three.

Pancakes are misunderstood and underappreciated. Maybe we overlook the poor pancake because it looks and tastes like a dessert. Pancakes by themselves are loaded with carbohydrates and are not high in fat or calories if you buy "complete" pancake mixes. Fruit, berries, and nuts can be added to make them more fun. Pancakes become sinful when we gob syrup and butter all over them. Totally skip the butter because all you taste is the butter and not the pancake. Use light syrup. Some of these syrups have a buttery flavor blended right in. These light syrups have improved in taste considerably in the last several years and are almost indistinguishable from regular syrup. Pancakes made with your personal touch may take a bit more time and certainly create more kitchen mess, so you may want to save them for weekend breakfasts and let the whole family pitch in with the preparation. Family members can take a turn on Sunday to create their version of the pancake breakfast—blueberries for Beth, bananas for Bobbie, nonfat sour cream for Dad, and apple pancakes for Mom.

Egg omelets using low-calorie and low-fat ingredients are great weekend breakfast foods. Making your omelets with egg whites only cuts down on the fat content. You can also cut down on the LDL cholesterol, which comes from the yolk, by using only half the yolks of the total amount of eggs you are using. So for a family of five if you are going to use a dozen eggs for all your omelets, separate out six of the egg yolks prior to whisking the eggs together in a bowl. Make ham omelets one Sunday, turkey sausage omelets the next, and so on.

Lunch: Taking your lunch to work and school is the best alternative. What you can make for yourself is just so much tastier than what you will get from the school cafeteria or a fast-food place near the office. Make lunches fun and attractive. Pack several varieties of foods, one of which should be a fruit serving. Always buy the light turkey, ham, chicken, or beef luncheon meat now available in most supermarkets. Remember to use wheat or grain bread, or use a tortilla and make a wrap. Make a pita sandwich by stuffing the pita bread with your favorite ingredients. Both pitas and tortillas are healthier alternatives than bread made with white flour. Add lettuce and tomato for a vegetable portion, and watch the condiments you use for taste. Rotate the variety of the lunch daily. This is easier than you may think. All of these tips will keep your family interested and excited about taking their lunch every day and will keep them away from the unhealthy stuff.

An interesting lunch can be made with low-fat ham, lettuce, tomato, olives, and parsley. Finely chop this mixture. Lightly sprinkle with rice vinegar and stuff this into a pita or wrap into a tortilla. This produces a healthy, low-calorie, low-fat lunch for the whole family.

Of course you are now eating such healthy and interesting food that leftovers are fun to take to work and school. With modern packaging and microwaves everywhere lunch can become a mini-dinner sampler. Be creative here. If you are using dinner leftovers, you may want to jazz them up a bit for a next-day lunch. Leftover chicken can be shredded while you are cleaning up after dinner and put into small containers. When you make lunches, just add nonfat mayonnaise and some chopped sweet pickles and in an instant you have chicken salad that can be eaten right out of the container or wrapped in a tortilla. Most meat can be used in a similar way.

Dinner: Dinner can be one of the most fun meals to make low calorie and low fat. There are so many products in the supermarket now that can help you with dinner. Some frozen prepared entrees are quite tasty and healthy. The Healthy Choice line of foods is good. These frozen low-calorie choices can be quite convenient during the week when you are trying to fit in your family activity during the evening. Another quick and healthy dinner alternative is frozen veggie burgers. They are quite tasty and make a solid dinner when paired with a salad, light soup, and multigrain bread.

A hint about dinner: The multigenerational style of eating many of us were raised with often overemphasized the entrée at dinner. Traditionally this entrée was the big fat and calorie culprit. Begin to change that tradition in your family. Prepare larger portions of healthy side dishes such as salads, steamed vegetables, and soups. Place larger portions of side dishes on the dinner plates. Cook limited amounts of meats. If family members are still hungry, give them no other alternative but to have more of these side dishes. Do not allow them to help themselves to the refrigerator to supplement or substitute for the meal you prepared. This only undercuts the healthy style you are trying to establish.

Dinner, like all of the meals in Family Fit, takes some investigation and you will come up with some surprising results. For example, one would think that an Italian beef sandwich is totally out of the question in a healthy diet. Surprise! Frozen Italian beef made on Italian bread has a low saturated fat content and is not high in calories. It is also high in protein and is a quick dinner for a family on a weeknight. Pair it with a light salad and a fruit dessert and you have a very healthy meal. Make sure you read the nutritional label on the type of frozen beef and the bread you buy, but these items, like some other foods you might not expect, are actually healthy choices for the family.

> ***Become a predator in the supermarket, not a consumer! Scrutinize labels, take nothing for granted, and take no prisoners. If it is not low calorie and low in saturated fat, let the store keep it!***

Eating Protests

Families often find themselves in unhealthy eating patterns because the adults in the family are unwilling to exert their leadership. Adults will give in to a child's gratifications because they are afraid to establish rules and boundaries with the child even though they know that the child's wants are unhealthy. This must stop if we are going to establish healthy lifestyles in our families and break this cycle of obesity. Chapter 9 will discuss strategies to help families set rules and boundaries with their children.

Mike and Maria Pena are upper-middle-class parents with a ten-year-old boy and an eight-year-old girl. Mike is the head of a Fortune 500 company. Mike comes home every night late from the office and sits down to a very healthy meal that Maria has prepared for him. Both Mike and Maria are trim, fit adults in their mid-thirties. Their children have eaten hours earlier and have the same exact meal every night—grilled cheddar cheese sandwiches on white bread and a glass of whole milk.

One evening, Mike happened to run into the family pediatrician at a social function and asked her why the children always seemed to have an inordinate number of minor illnesses. They had a long discussion trying to figure out possible rationales for the frequency of the children's sicknesses. Finally, Mike asked Dr. Jones whether the children's nutrition could have something to do with their sickliness. When Dr. Jones learned that the kids ate grilled cheese sandwiches every night, tater tots at every lunch, and chocolaty cereal every morning for breakfast without fail, she was appalled. She immediately asked if they were taking multivitamins.

Mike lamented, "We can't get them to take anything. We try, but they refuse and then they have the most terrible temper tantrums you can imagine."

Dr. Jones correctly confronted Mike on letting the children control the parents, especially on something so important as nourishment.

Mike, seemingly helpless, shrugged. "But how can we get them to change?"

With that, Dr. Jones shot back, "You cook what you cook for them and they eat it and that's all!"

"And if they don't eat?" Mike asked.

"Then they don't eat. Or try a little of my mother's intervention. They don't leave the table until they eat what you prepared," Dr. Jones answered.

"But they could be there all evening," Mike felt compelled to point out, still helpless.

"Yep," is all Dr. Jones said.

That real-life conversation illustrates how parents abdicate to their children even in the face of unhealthy choices they make for themselves. As ridiculous as it seems, that scene is played out many times in our families. Parents must take more control over health decisions for their children. If they protest or complain or throw a tantrum, *so what?* You are the adult and you know what is best for them. Stick with your new Family Fit Program. Their complaining will die down as they see you are going to be relentless and not give in to their whines.

Snacking and Multimeal Programs

Like multivitamins, snacking is controversial in nutrition circles. Snacks or several light meals are being trumpeted as a newly discovered, healthier alternative to eating than the traditional three meals per day. The adherents to the multimeal theory claim that small meals keep hunger down and increase metabolism so more calories are burned and fewer are consumed overall. There are several cautions to be considered before a family adopts the multimeal plan. Several small meals daily make it harder for families to control what is being consumed at those meals, particularly in youngsters. This increases tremendously the likelihood of departing from the Family Fit plan. It appears to be no coincidence that these multimeal plans seem to have developed in this day and age when families are so busy. Is it coincidental that families are spending less time together, coming home later, and now need to eat more times each day away from each other? The multimeal plan increases the tendency to eat apart from our families rather than letting meals bring families closer together as in the Family Fit Program.

The multimeal plan also makes eating more work. Most of these programs want your family to eat six small meals each day. That means you have to prepare, plan, and clean up after three more meals each day, and multiply that by each family member. Food doesn't become fun; it becomes a bigger burden. This negative attitude toward food propels you right back into the cycle of obesity.

Take a look at the times when the typical family will eat their meals. Let's estimate that breakfast will be typically 7:00 a.m., lunch between 11:00 a.m. and 1:00 p.m., and dinner approximately 7:00 p.m., and the longest time between meals is six hours. Considering that digestion is a slow process and that we are eating better than ever in the Family Fit plan, this amount of time is not an intolerable wait between meals. Furthermore, add the increased physical activity that the Family Fit Program calls for and you will find that metabolism will be increased automatically by participating in this program. In the Family Fit Program you will not have to depend on your food to increase your metabolism.

Keep in mind that if you feel hunger pains, this could be **dehydration** as mentioned previously. Drink plenty of water throughout the day and you may find that your habit of requiring a snack will diminish.

Similarly, you will note from the Family Day Planner that snacking is not a part of the Family Fit Program. Snacks are dangerous because they tend to be spontaneous and do not apply forward thinking. Snacking also adds calories onto your daily intake. As a result of these added calories, do you skimp on something at meals to lower your total calorie count for the day? This type of habit can break up the rhythm of the Family Fit Program. If your body seems to crave food between meals, and this will differ from person to person, then have something ready that is very low in calories and high in nutrients. The Slim Fast bars mentioned previously can be a good choice; so can fruit.

> **HEALTHY SNACKS TO HAVE ON HAND**
> - Fruit
> - Dried fruit
> - Raw vegetables
> - Energy bars, but be careful here; read labels
> - Natural fruit juices
> - Low-fat/low-calorie crackers, bagel chips, etc.

But snacking is so unpredictable; anything you carry with you that is fresh may be wasted because you didn't need a snack that day.

A final word on snacking: Snacking is often a learned behavior rather than a need. The Family Fit Program is all about learning a new lifestyle away from obesity and obese behavior. Try to resist the urge to snack as a part of your Family Fit commitment.

Snacking can lead back to bad habits.

It's possible that snacking has trained your mind that you must have this food right now. Be careful and try not to snack. The danger for those that get into the snack habit is that one day you may not have a nutritious alternative, and you will cheat.

THINGS TO REMEMBER:
- Develop new eating habits—40-40-20.
- Know and monitor your number of calories each day.
- Understand how to calculate calories for your basal metabolic rate (BMR, see page 104).
- Eliminate as much fat from your diet as you can.
- Make food and eating fun.
- Drink more water.
- Avoid snacking if possible.

CHAPTER SIX

The Second Way—Motivating Generations to Change

Motivation to change is a field of human behavior that has often been studied. Unfortunately, very little of this vast amount of information has been applied in the field of obesity. When motivation is discussed, it is glossed over or, at best, simple external rewards are pointed out to keep people on their diets. External rewards have their place in motivating people to change, but they are only a small part of the larger picture of how motivation can be applied to obesity. Similarly, motivation is not a person running around in sequined shorts screaming at people to not be fat. There is a large, sophisticated body of scientific studies on motivation.

The leader in the field of motivation studies is the business world. Business has long recognized that motivating employees to be more productive is pivotal to industry success. Why weight loss hasn't given motivation this same prominence is a mystery and may be another reason why so many weight loss programs have not stood the test of time.

Weight loss programs or lifestyle change programs are not alone in neglecting the power of motivation techniques to enact change and success. Family life has also been lacking application of motivation techniques to help family members live a more fulfilling, healthier lifestyle.

Recognizing the importance of motivation in the goal of changing to a healthier lifestyle can reap great rewards for family success. In the Family Fit Program, motivation is one of the three pillars of the program along with Diet/Nutrition and Activity. Because motivation techniques are such powerful tools and because a more thorough application of them is new to both family lifestyle change and to weight loss, application of motivation techniques will result in success in a short period of time. The use of the motivation techniques outlined here is one of the prime reasons why the Family Fit Program can boast that the family will see success in three weeks.

The groundwork for motivating your family has been laid both in preparing for the program (Chapter Four) and changing how we approach food (Chapter Five). The way we talk about food, as discussed in Chapter Four, is key to how we motivate our family members. Our words fill the environment around our homes with our philosophy on life. Our family members pick up this philosophy not by having us sit down with them and giving them a lecture, but by hearing the words we speak daily that convey our approach to life. Surrounding people in an environment that gives consistent messages about a philosophy is one of the most powerful motivational techniques used in the business world. This concept is called *affirmation*.

Use Affirmations

An affirmation is the transmission of positive messages through the use of subtle methods in the person's surroundings. Do you have some pens at home with your company's logo? That's an affirmation. Do you wear a polo shirt with your company's name on it? Again, that is an affirmation. At your place of business are there signs that have motivational messages on them, such as "Work is Pride" or "59 days without an accident" or "The friendly place to work"? These are all affirmations that leave a subliminal message in your mind that you should do your best on the job or you should like this as a place to work.

Do these affirmations work? Big business would not spend millions on these pens, notebooks, logos, signs, and clothing if they didn't. Consider the company where you work. Do you think the powers that be would spend a nickel on any of this unless they received a return on their investment? Convinced?

Don't confuse pure advertisements with affirmations. The purpose of advertising is to compel you to buy a product or service. The purpose of affirmations is to compel you to act in a certain way. Advertisements can be affirmations, but effective affirmations are always powerful subliminal messages, which motivate people to act in a certain way. Not all advertisements are subliminal. They are often direct manipulations.

Now, let's look at how you can use affirmation around your home to motivate your family. Remember, how we talk about eating and food is one of our biggest avenues for sending out affirmations to keep up with the program. Should you put up big signs and banners printed with motivational mantras? Well, maybe you should. But in most homes such banners may clash with the sofa. How about a sign on the refrigerator instead? Why not make it a big "Family Fit"? Or maybe a sticky note on the lunch you make for a family member? Or try a big family calendar somewhere that merges the Family Day Planner on the specific days of the week for these three weeks? Display this Family Day Planner/calendar prominently in the house. Underneath the days of the week write in red ink, "Way to Go, Everyone!" and/or "Keep it up!" "I'm proud of you, Lamar!!!" "Nice workout today, Bill!" "Super supper, Mom!" Be creative, be corny, be bold, and be confident…but be. People are motivated by seeing and hearing positive affirmations.

Step into most young people's bedrooms and you will see posters celebrating a musician, sports figure, or some other idol. How about buying those kids a poster that affirms the lifestyle you are trying to establish? How about an artistic rendition of a philosopher saying something positive about health? Go out and buy one for your children. Or paste up articles you read in magazines or the newspaper that promote a healthy lifestyle. Put a note on them for the family to see: "Did you all see this? We're on the road to a better life! Mom."

You may run across an article that talks about a healthy food product you just discovered. Pass it around the family. *People* magazine writes about how Julia Roberts jumps rope every day to stay in shape. Make sure everyone in the family sees it. These actions surround the family in the message you want delivered. And don't worry if teenage Marcus just glances at the article and passes it to the next person. The message is still being transmitted.

The use of affirmations is one of the most powerful motivational tools. Think about how you can apply affirmations and use them generously around your household.

Motivate Others

The second most powerful motivator is person-to-person motivation. The most disenfranchised, unmotivated, angry, hopeless individual becomes positively affected when someone comes up to him, looks him in the eye, and says, "Good job, I'm proud of you!"

Avoid Negative Reinforcement

That human contact rewarding the person for a good effort is priceless. Always be positive, even in the face of failure or setback. If a family member slips up in the program, don't tear her down; build her up and look positively at the experience. This is not a part of your nature? You weren't raised this way? Well, that's why those old ways contributed to the cycle of obesity. They didn't work very well. Negative reinforcement or negative statements are the worst form of motivation. People do not respond when you are yelling at them or being critical. They shut down and they don't hear any message. So save your breath. Negative, hostile, critical messages are a waste of your words.

Negative statements are not motivational.

What is the best thing to say after a failure or a mistake? Try, "Well, okay, you messed up. Now, what did you learn from that? Don't forget. One mistake is not the ruin of the whole program. It's just one moment in the program. Pick yourself up and get back on track. Just think of how well you've done up until that moment. You can do it again. We're all behind you." Think about how much better that is than something like, "Well, you messed up. Now you have to start all over again." Or "Jimmy is doing so much better than you—now you really have a lot of catching up to do. You'd better work harder!" Or "Jeez, don't do that again." All of these statements are possibly meant well, but they all have a negative spin on them.

While your family is on the Family Fit Program, make sure you give thousands of positive "I'm proud of you," "Great job," "Nice way to handle that," "Great workout," "Thanks for being with me today," "Wonderful meal," or "I love you" statements. And include another thousand statements that compliment how your family members look, such as: "You're looking buff" and "Looking great, keep it up." And when you compliment another's looks, don't be afraid to be bold. "Your spare tire is really getting flat! I can see a big difference." Or "Your thighs are toning up." This is very important and powerful in motivation. You may not be able to do something like this with someone outside of the family, but with family members statements that go to the heart of physical problems they are concerned about can be powerful statements of affirmation, propelling family members onward with their goals. The motivating force of your statement will vibrate through the loved one and inside he will appreciate it. What's more, when you do bring up the "forbidden" area, you are letting the family member know that you are concerned and paying close attention to his or her Family Fit Program.

All of these person-to-person statements are powerful motivators that nothing you can buy can replace. Hopefully, this habit of complimenting each other and the good feeling it generates will continue in your family.

Along with positive statements and acknowledgments of another's performance, *modeling* is a very powerful motivator.

> *If you want your family to act in a certain way, you must model those actions yourself.*

Become a Role Model
Modeling is one of the most effective methods of bringing along a family member who may be lagging in the program or even reluctant to join in. If these family members are continually bombarded with models of a new healthy lifestyle, you will see an increase in their motivation to come aboard.

The third best motivator is the positive reward that comes from within. When we do things that make us feel good, that accomplishment is a huge reward and motivator. We are motivated when what we do is fun and interesting and we can feel some degree of success at it. Many social scientists have called this self-reward, self-motivation, or a sense of mastery.

Let's take a look at how this develops in young people. During the typical hectic morning rush at the Johnson house one day, the vacuum cleaner broke down as Mr. Johnson was heading into the shower. Mrs. Johnson asked him if he would try to fix it before he went to work. Strained for time, Mr. Johnson agreed, but his voice betrayed the stress of an extra obligation that would make him late for work. Taking in this whole scene, five-year-old Justin asked Mom if he could fix the vacuum cleaner while Dad was in the shower. Thinking how cute this offer was coming from her five-year-old little man of the house, Mom agreed, never in her wildest imagination thinking it would do any more harm, or good for that matter. By the time Dad came out of the shower, Justin turned on the vacuum, and by some weird twist of fate, it worked! It didn't matter whether Justin kicked the vacuum and dislodged something stuck; the important thing was that the vacuum was working. Mom was ecstatic and Dad was too because he could get to work on time. As for Justin, his chest stuck out as if he had an iron lung, and he had a smile from ear to ear. Justin was proud of his effort and his accomplishment, no matter how serendipitous it was. From that moment on Justin became known in the house as "the little fix-it man." Well into his twenties, whenever anything needed fixing, setting up, or a trip to the repair shop, you can bet that Justin was the guy to do it in the Johnson home.

This is the classic development of motivation to do a task in a family. This same type of scene can take place in your household around fitness and a healthy lifestyle. Let one of the young people lead the family in an activity. Let another take charge of preparing a meal. Do these things not as an assignment but as part of the fun, with a sense of mastery. If a young person, old person, spouse, or friend has a role in the Family Fit Program, they will be extra-motivated to perform and lead the others. People become disenfranchised when they feel they have no place or role in the whole endeavor. People of the older generations in particular drop out because of this sense of not having a meaningful role. Give Grandma and Grandpa the task of getting to your house each morning for the morning activity (see the Family Day Planner) and making sure the activity starts on time. Do that and they'll never be late, nor will your activity. Give each family member an essential role and you will see motivation skyrocket.

One of the best ways to develop self-motivation is to have a cause that you are passionate about. A personal cause drives a person to put extraordinary energy into endeavors. One of the most outstanding features of the program is that it brings families together by focusing on a need or want that the vast majority of people of *all* ages want desperately for themselves—to be healthy and to look good.

> *Being healthy is vital to people of all ages. Because of this, nothing can pull your family together better than a healthy lifestyle, healthy eating, and fitness.*

This statement is so important and true. Nothing will draw the attention of each family member, no matter from what generation, as well as health and fitness. For that reason, installing the Family Fit Program in your family will generate a great deal of its own motivation. Think about it. Adults of parenting age are vitally concerned about the health and well-being of their families. Children love activity and quality time with their family, and they love eating and being focused on food. Teens are greatly centered on their bodies and how they look. Research shows that the two biggest concerns of adults in the senior years are their health and food. Looking at the critical issues of all these age groups, you couldn't dream of a better focus than the elements of the Family Fit Program. Using the motivation techniques here will just add to the fire already burning inside each family member to be healthy and to look and feel great.

By planting the Family Fit Program in your family, you will be directing them to a personal cause that will feed internal motivation. Once each family member can see the visible results of living this healthier lifestyle, they all will be focused and will continue with their motivation to change.

When motivating family members, you must recognize what doesn't work as much as what does work. What is the worst form of motivation? The least effective techniques for motivating someone to change use external pressure and guilt. The old phrase "Don't do it for someone else; do it for yourself" couldn't be more accurate. If a person is forcing you to do something, you may go along for a short duration, but your motivation is not coming from within. As soon as the other person removes the pressure, you will stop what you are doing. In short, you can get someone to participate, but you are not building a lifestyle change that will last over the course of his or her life.

Lead by Example

The Harrises were a typical family—two adults living with their two teenage children. Dad Frank had been an athlete all his life and worked out daily. Mom Cara was never athletic nor had she ever worked out. Their daughter Camie was also not athletic and had little interest in exercise. Their son Tim was an athlete from the time he was born. He played soccer, baseball, tennis, and football; he biked, he ran, he swam. He would try anything that was physical. This close-knit family had to adjust family time for Dad's runs or health club time. When Tim was old enough to play on sports teams, they all went to his games.

Frank and Tim never prodded or pushed Cara and Camie to become more physically active. After a few years of this split in the family, Cara accompanied Frank to the health club one day because they had a social event right after Frank's workout. While waiting for Frank to finish his workout, Cara mistakenly signed up for an introductory aerobics class. She thought she was signing up for something completely different—a heart checkup that sounded like a deal at $25. The day before the class began, a very enthusiastic staff person from the health club called Cara to confirm her class time. The staff person reminded Cara to bring appropriate workout clothes. Still thinking this was a heart checkup, Cara didn't blink an eye at this request.

Cara went to the introductory program, which turned out to be a cardio-fitness class employing step-aerobics and kickboxing. She loved it and was hooked. Cara began to attend the health club classes with a furor that surpassed even Frank. After months of being surrounded by three physically active family members, Camie began to go to the club as well. Camie likes the aerobic dance classes, and although she doesn't exercise nearly as much as her family members do, she still consistently works out at least three days each week.

The Harrises illustrate how effective sound motivational techniques work in a family. No one pressured Cara and Camie. There was no begging or bartering for health club visits. Still, all the family members blended into a lifestyle of regular physical activity.

Be Patient

It may take some patience with one or more family members, as it did in the Harris household, but if we surround our family members in a positive lifestyle that works and don't give up, they will come around.

For the same reason that pressure and guilt don't work, bribes simply do not work as motivation. Do not use them in this program. If you find yourself saying to a family member, "I'll buy you that new pair of jeans you wanted if you just come along with us on Sunday," you have failed and have lost money in the process. Will the family member go on Sunday? Probably, but what have you gained?

With all of this discussion of motivation, you may be wondering why material rewards haven't been mentioned yet. That's because being rewarded with material things is not a very powerful human motivator. This may come as a surprise to many. This is not to say that rewards cannot be used to motivate family members, but there is a time and place for such rewards, and they shouldn't be the highlight of your motivational system while participating in Family Fit. It can be quite rewarding to buy special workout clothes for everyone prior to starting the program. This makes family members feel good, but these clothes will quickly be old. This is exactly what happens with any material reward. It gets old, and then the family is looking for the next reward. Even the richest family may run out of either money or ideas of what to buy next to keep the family motivated. Again, material rewards help motivate in small ways, but they pale in comparison to the more powerful techniques of the atmosphere you surround the family in, your person-to-person positive affirmation, and the internal cause that is being built.

Be Genuine
A word of caution about our language when we use person-to-person encouragement: It is vital to the success of this motivational technique to keep it genuine. Do not patronize or heap false praise on a family member. People of all generations see through false praise, but for young people in particular false praise or patronization is like nails on a chalkboard. They will shudder inside when you subject them to this. These words will work against you and take the family member away from participating rather than motivating them onward.

Here is where blunt honesty is critical. If Grandma shows up for family activity in a T-shirt that is much too tight, do not compliment her on how much trimmer she looks in that shirt. Be honest. "Gram, you're looking so much better, but I don't think you're quite ready for *that* shirt. You may be more comfortable doing our exercises in something bigger, but I bet in another week or so, that shirt is going to work fine."

Becoming a family motivator may take a change in your attitude as a parent. You may need to rethink the negative ways you use to try to get your family to do things. You will need to incorporate a positive approach and become a leader, model, and mentor for your family. Isn't that what parenting is all about?

In the following pages we provide ideas in which you can motivate the family to participate in the Family Fit approach. Remember, much scientific evidence has shown that these are the most powerful methods around. You may hear about some tips from an e-mail or a magazine, which can help in some minor ways, but keep your focus on the broader techniques listed here and success will surely come.

> **THINGS TO REMEMBER:**
> - Make the program interesting and fun.
> - Speak in ways that motivate—positively.
> - Use affirmations all the time.
> - Give person-to-person reinforcement.
> - Heap praise on the family liberally.
> - Give honest feedback constantly.
> - Use material rewards sparingly.
> - Allow family members to gain mastery over the program.
> - Be a model of what you want your family to do.

CHAPTER SEVEN

The Third Way—Family Fitness Activity

Mention exercise, and many of us cringe. The word *exercise* has evolved to evoke the image of some enormous white elephant that we just can't get off our backs. We picture in our heads our bodies sweating and straining while we move in some contorted way for an hour or more.

These images are precisely why so many people have difficulty keeping exercise as a part of their daily lifestyle. We hold this mistaken notion that if we don't exercise in that way, we aren't deriving any benefit from the effort. All of this is false. The image is false, the thinking is false, and the approach is false.

Just Do It

The most important part of exercise is to just go and do it. There is nothing wrong with just getting on your exercise clothes and "being in the moment" with exercise. Consider it a victory if you just allocate the time, change your clothes, and show up. *Go easy on yourself.* Just the act of showing up for an activity is a vitally important first step toward success in the Family Fit Program. In addition, showing up has great side effects. What a break in the routine of the day. What a stress reliever. Change clothes, move your body around. When people start with this, the rest comes easy. Encourage all family members to just show up in the same fashion.

Adult family members do youngsters a great service by this act of showing up on a regular basis in the Family Fit Program. Nowhere does the Family Fit Program ask adults to be fitness fanatics; instead, allocate the time and be there for your family. You are then installing fitness as a part of your family's lifestyle. What a wonderful gift to give your children!

Put on the sweat clothes and walk once around the street where you live at a brisk pace. Do that every morning, increasing the pace you walk at, the distance, or both every other day. Do just this and you will be ahead of all the others who are not getting up off the couch because they don't have the time to do a four-mile run. They can wait forever, but the street won't come to them—they have to go to the street.

Forget About Workouts and Exercise

It is this conception of exercise that has led us to use the term *activity* instead of *exercise* in the Family Fit Program. This is important particularly in a program that includes participants whose ages span several generations.

Older generations have often held the biggest misconceptions about exercise, and only recently have small percentages of seniors incorporated light exercise into their lifestyles. To broadcast the term *exercise* as a pillar of this program is a sure way to scare off senior family members whom we are actively embracing as key participants in this program. Many sedentary young people will have the same attitude toward exercise as seniors do.

Using the term *activity* is more descriptive of this pillar anyway. Activity can encompass the fitness goals of the beginner as well as the advanced fitness enthusiast. This is the goal of this pillar. It is designed to satisfy any member of the family and to do this while the family participates together as much as possible. Let's take a look at how this is done.

We approach the activity pillar of Family Fit by first dispelling some misconceptions about including the whole family in physical activity together.

First, young people and adults can work out together, and the adult can meet his or her fitness goals no matter what they are.

Second, children should be included in family activities from birth.

Third, young people should be welcome in health clubs and the YMCA as long as they are supervised closely by their parent(s), follow the rules of the club, do not disturb others using the club, and learn club etiquette.

Fourth, it is not true that unconventional workouts that involve physical movement and aerobic activity are just playtime and have no fitness benefit.

Fifth, family members of all ages can participate and benefit by strength training geared to their level.

Sixth, seniors, regardless of physical limitation, should be included in the physical activity that the whole family is engaged in.

Seventh, there is always time for physical activity in the day.

Mom (Tina), Dad (Jim), Grandpa Bill, Grandma Jane, and the kids, Joey, Kim, and little Billy Barnes, are one week into their Family Fit Program. Tina and Jim have run marathons and regularly run about 35 miles each week. Grandpa Bill uses a walker because of a stroke he suffered some years ago. With all this potential limitation, this family has embraced and is successful in being active together.

There is a park one-quarter mile from the Barnes's home. They start their activity time by walking briskly to the park. Grandpa Bill follows with his walker as fast as he can go. No one worries that he is behind or that they have to wait a few minutes for him to arrive. This activity time is not about competition. The Barnes's activity time is also about honesty, and everyone else walks faster than Grandpa does. He's okay with that, and so is everyone else. In fact, on most days Joey and Kim hold a mock race to get to the park, so they arrive first. Tina and Jim walk fast but not at breakneck speed, and they arrive next. Grandma Jane walks with Billy and they arrive at a casual but serious pace after that, and not too far behind the parade is Grandpa, moving quite spryly with his walker.

Once in the park, Tina and Jim almost immediately take off on a run around the perimeter of the park. One lap around the park is two miles, and while Tina and Jim run, they can see the rest of the family making their way toward the center of the park. After three laps around the park, Tina and Jim jog slowly to wherever the rest of the family has stopped.

On this day, Grandma, Grandpa, Joey, Kim, and Billy play a brisk game of soccer. Grandpa is the goalie, and it's the boys against the girls, each twosome taking turns on offense and defense. Grandpa can't jump, move to his left with lightning speed, or dive for a shot on goal, so many of the shots aimed in his direction end up as scores for that team. So what? We repeat, this activity is not about competition. No one remembers the scores of these games anyway. Grandpa is lightning-quick with his hands after forty-five years of being a pipefitter, so if the ball is kicked right at him, he's going to bat it away. He always grins from ear to ear when that happens, and it seems to happen often in these games. Tina and Jim join this raucous match, each taking the appropriate side. While the kids and Grandma continue with the rhythm of their game, Tina and Jim pause frequently to stretch their muscles from their run.

After a short period of this intense activity, they all walk slowly back home. On most days they walk together in one big group engaged in a hearty conversation.

No one can say that everyone in this multigenerational family isn't meeting their fitness needs. For Tina and Jim, this time with their family takes no more time than if they went out for a run on their own. For Grandma and Grandpa, they can be as physically active as their bodies will allow. And the children are learning at a young age how to incorporate physical activity into their day.

This same family scene can take place within a variety of physical activities. The Barnes family provides another good example of this while participating in a very different kind of activity.

On the days that the Barnes family does not do aerobic activity, they do strength training to build and tone the muscles. Tina and Jim bought an inexpensive weight set some years ago. Each family member takes a turn using a dumbbell or barbell to tone a body part. Grandma uses the lightest weights with her arms. Grandpa can't bend to grab his weights, so another family member instantly becomes his spotter and gets the weight he requests. Grandpa typically works his large arms and shoulders to keep them in shape for balancing on the walker. He always does some leg lifts with medium-heavy weights in hopes of gaining some more power in his damaged limbs. Jim and Tina work out with heavy weights to keep their legs and upper bodies in the best of shape for running.

A totally different activity, yet each family member is included in a meaningful way. This latter scene could easily be taking place in a health club or gym. It emphasizes that the Family Fit Program creates workout partners from your family members. What better workout partners could you have than your family members?

By the way, many exercise researchers are urging weight training for all age groups. Studies have shown that even ninety-year-olds develop greater confidence and are less likely to fall and hurt themselves after starting a weight training program. Strengthening muscles leads to strengthening bones, which prevents osteoporosis. Muscle cells use more energy than fat cells. Well-toned muscles burn excess calories in the body. Weight training also increases metabolism, so more calories are burned even when at rest. Weight training is a fitness activity that is easy to adapt to any age group and lends itself well to generation-spanning family participation. An ideal weight training session is twenty minutes long, with two to three sessions per week to build muscles and keep them toned. Weight training can fit perfectly into the segments outlined in the Family Day Planner. See Chapter Four.

From the examples given so far in this chapter, we see this family has participated in the same type of activity together, and each person was able to work at his or her own level while still participating with the family. There are many physical activities that will adapt to the specific level of different age groups. Swimming comes to mind almost immediately, but swimming is not readily available for many families. You may want to save swimming for one of the weekend activity days because by the time your family drives to a pool, changes, swims, changes again, and then drives home, you have quite a time expenditure.

Go for a Walk

Another marvelous fitness activity that the entire family can participate in *and* that is very accessible and *time sensitive* is walking. Walking is a terrific fitness activity for the whole family, and exercise physiologists are coming out with new research that suggests walking may be the best overall exercise there is, bar none. Some of these scientists are so excited about the benefits of walking that they are touting it as the *perfect* exercise. One scientist said that if everyone were to walk briskly for thirty minutes a day, the incidence of chronic diseases could be cut by as much as 40 percent. If you walk briskly for at least three to four hours over the course of a week, this has the same effect as fifteen to twenty minutes of more vigorous exercise done each day in that week. A twelve-year study of sixty- to eighty-year-olds demonstrates that daily, moderately intense, two-mile walks cut the death rate for these individuals in half!

There is no question that the benefits of walking are increasingly being uncovered. Yet, walking gets slighted as a valuable fitness activity probably because of the same mind-set described at the beginning of this chapter. People have developed a preconceived notion about walking so they don't do it, thinking it has little value. Paradoxically, using this thinking, they opt to do no fitness activity. Go figure.

A fitness activity time for the whole family doesn't have to be made up of just one activity for everyone to participate in. The trip to the health club is a good example here. One person can be taking an aerobics class while two others swim, a fourth is weight training, and the fifth is doing circuit training. By being at the club together, everybody will cross with everyone else with plenty of time to check in with each other. This is still time together right out of the guidelines of the Family Day Planner.

The bottom line to your family fitness activity time is that the whole family is participating in a physical activity. Ideally, this activity is one that the whole family can enjoy, but there may be times when several family members are doing different activities from the others at the same time and in the same space. Sometimes these times of divergence make for more family interaction as family members talk afterward about their workouts.

On page 152, we provide a chart that lists suggestions for activities that a family can participate in together. Each activity lists any age adaptation it may require, where it will fit into the Family Day Planner, (long, short, or moderate duration), and any variations needed from its traditional participation to include family members of any age. These activities on the list are just suggestions and are not meant to be an exhaustive list of the many activities your family can participate in. Because there can be so many variations of activities, a Family Planner is also presented after this list. Use the planner with your family to think up your own varieties of fitness activities. The idea here is to have fun, be creative, and get out there and be active together.

This list dramatically highlights the wide variety of fitness activities that the family can easily participate in together. How can any family say that they don't have time to do some of these? The beauty of incorporating an activity into the day (see Family Day Planner) is that it makes your day more efficient in the long run. Why? Most parents want to spend some quality time with their children throughout the day. We all accept the importance of this. With Family Fit a part of your family life, this quality family time is built right into the activity time. The Family Day Planner clearly shows that you create your family time, you meet your adult fitness needs, and you create more individual time for yourself, all by doing something that the whole family will enjoy and benefit from.

> *A family fitness activity is a great opportunity to spend quality family time with family members of all ages.*

There are still a couple of footnotes to be added to this list of activities. Your family should *always* include *warm-up, cooldown,* and *stretching* in every activity. Look back at the story of the Barnes family going to the park. Their walk to the park is their warm-up and their walk home is their cooldown. They incorporated stretching as a part of the activity. These movements are very critical for the body. They allow the muscles to stay healthy, and they prevent muscle cramping and muscle ache. The importance of these movements cannot be stressed enough. For family members of all ages these three parts of the activity prevent injury. Including these in your Family Fit Program teaches young family members a great lesson in health and fitness at an early age and puts them ahead of other kids their age.

> *Always include a warm-up, cooldown, and stretch as a part of every activity.*

FAMILY FITNESS ACTIVITIES

Activity*	What's Involved	Equipment
Aerobics (home)	Rapid body movements; some coordination	Video
Aerobics classes (club/gym)	Rapid body movements; some coordination	Appropriate clothing
Badminton	Hand-eye coordination; rapid body movements	Badminton set, yard space
Baseball	Hand-eye coordination; timing	Space, bat, ball, glove
Basketball	Coordination; strength	Hoop, ball, space
Bowling	Coordination; spatial relations	Bowling alley, ball, pins, shoes
Cross-country skiing	Coordination; endurance	Skis, snow, space
Cycling	Coordination; endurance	Bikes, helmet (Recumbent bike for seniors)
Downhill skiing	Coordination; learned skill	Skis, handicap skis, helmet
Football	Coordination; strength and skill level; game knowledge	Football, space
Frisbee	Game knowledge; hand-eye coordination	Frisbee, space
Golf	Hand-eye coordination; patience	Clubs, golf course
Hiking	Strength; endurance	Shoes, clothing
Ice Skating	coordination; skill	Skates, rink
Jump rope	Coordination; endurance	Rope, space

*Always include a warm-up, cooldown, and stretch as part of every activity.

Day Planner Fit	Variation/Benefits
All durations	Great choice for home activity if the weather is bad; short timeframe; watch video together
Moderate	Would be ideal to get clubs to blend in multigenerations at same class
All durations	Fun, vigorous activity for all
Longer duration	Adjust pace
Moderate duration	Adjust pace
Longer duration	None
Longer duration	Handicap skis
Longer duration	Adjust speed
Very long duration	Adjust speed
All durations	Adjust pace of game
All durations	If slow/chaotic, make sure you make it more vigorous
Very long duration	Adjust skill/pace level
Longer duration	Adjust pace
Longer duration (travel to ice factor)	Good activity if you can get to rink or ice
Quick	Patience with young children

FAMILY FITNESS ACTIVITIES

Activity*	What's Involved	Equipment
Martial arts	Coordination; concentration	Instructor
Ping-Pong	Hand-eye coordination	Table, paddles and ball, space
Racquetball	Hand-eye coordination; endurance; knowledge of game; speed, agility	Racquet, balls, court
Handball/Squash	Hand-eye coordination; endurance; knowledge of game; speed/ability	Racquet, balls, court
Isometrics	Concentration; strength	None
Rollerblading	Coordination; balance	Roller blades, helmet, padding, space
Running	Strong limbs	Shoes, space
Tag games	Agility; speed	None
Tennis	Hand-eye coordination; strength; endurance; agility	Racquet, balls
Stair climbing	Endurance; strength	Shoes
Strength bands	Strength	Bands

*Always include a warm-up, cooldown, and stretch as part of every activity.

Day Planner Fit	Variation/Benefits
Very long duration	Must attend together; great if you have the time
All durations	A good workout that you can make vigorous
Moderate/long duration	Fun alternative
Moderate/long duration	Fun alternative
All durations	Very effective; all levels can participate at once; no need for special equipment or room, but buy a good manual and learn to do it correctly
All durations	May be difficult to impossible for some
Quick	Experienced runner may have to go out again/run with a stroller
All durations	Can be a real workout and include youngest children; make it vigorous by dodging/weaving
Moderate duration	Experienced/skilled players play on one court, others on the next
All durations	A great workout and you can find stairs everywhere
All durations	An inexpensive way to include strength training in the whole program; this can stand by itself or be added on to another activity to increase value

FAMILY FITNESS ACTIVITIES

Activity*	What's Involved	Equipment
Stretching	Concentration	Comfortable clothing
Swimming	Coordination; strength; skill	Pool, goggles
Volleyball	Hand-eye coordination. Strength. Game knowledge	Ball, net, space
Walking	Endurance	Shoes, space
Water aerobics	Coordination; concentration	Pool, swimwear
Weight training	Strength; coordination	Weights, spotters
Yoga	Flexibility; concentration	Mat

*Always include a warm-up, cooldown, and stretch as part of every activity.

Day Planner Fit	Variation/Benefits
All durations	A great activity that can stand by itself and should be included in every activity; a great fallback if stuck for ideas and time
Longer duration (travel to pool factor)	Advanced swimmers swim, others do water exercise/play
All durations	If game is slow/more stationary, make yourself get more vigorous
All durations	Walk in an area where all can view each other so faster walkers can go at their own pace
Longer duration (travel to pool factor)	None—all can do this great activity; some ages/skills will be more vigorous than others
All durations	An important part of a total fitness program all ages can do; before attempting weight training, talk to a trainer or get a thorough guide that explains how to use without causing injury
All durations	A great activity that can accommodate all ages

FAMILY PLANNER—ACTIVITIES

Activity							Planned For

_____		_____
_____		_____
_____		_____
_____		_____
_____		_____
_____		_____
_____		_____
_____		_____
_____		_____
_____		_____
_____		_____
_____		_____
_____		_____
_____		_____
_____		_____
_____		_____
_____		_____

Day Planner Fit

Feedback

Some final thoughts on these activities: A great way to satisfy all family members is to combine two or more of these fitness activities into a single activity. While younger family members are playing a game of tag, for example, the adults can be doing isometrics and some strength training with bands. All kinds of variations are possible. The important thing is for the adults not to make the excuse that you can't get your fitness needs met while you are participating with the kids or the seniors. *You can*, and you can do this efficiently and strenuously if that is your desire.

> ***Adults should not make the excuse that they are too advanced to participate at the same time that their youngest and oldest family members are also participating in a fitness activity. This is false.***

This old excuse has not only blocked adults from including these other family members in their fitness activity, but also has led to a decrease in quality family time available to families.

There is no doubt that those adults who have been training for many years may have to spice up their fitness activity time while participating with family members of all generations. This is very easy to accomplish. In many of the activities that your family will choose, these advanced adults will just have to be more vigorous than the activity demands. For example, if you are playing badminton with the family, make sure you are running after the birdie when it goes out of bounds. Run to change sides. Dart around to back up a play. Play like a little ferret. Don't just stand there and wait for the birdie to hit you in the nose. As Grandma and Grandpa or cousin Tom walks back from the yard to the house, do some sprints, or go for your daily run while they baby-sit the kids for a few minutes. Think and plan your activity time out *for yourself.* And be flexible in your thinking. If you move like that little ferret on a double cappuccino during a game you are not used to playing, you will be surprised at the huffing and puffing you'll do, even if you ran a marathon last year. Try it.

> **THINGS TO REMEMBER:**
> - Just show up.
> - All ages are active together.
> - There is always time for physical activity in the day.
> - Unconventional activities can be a great workout.
> - Have fun with your activities.
> - Always include a warm-up, cooldown, and stretching.

PART IV
STAYING ON THE PROGRAM

CHAPTER EIGHT

Triggers That Lead Back to Bad Habits

This chapter will briefly describe the common situations that will trigger family members into thoughts and behaviors that may jettison them back into habits that will put them right back into the cycle of obesity. Warning! These triggers will be everywhere. They are unavoidable. The first defense against falling victim to these triggers is to recognize that they are out there trying to lure us back into obesity.

Work and School Cafeterias

Now cafeterias are serving Taco Bell, McDonald's, and other fast-food products right in workplaces and schools. Your family will pass these high temples of fat and calories while taking a break from the stress of the day. The association of these unhealthy foods with the relaxation of the lunch period may be too overpowering.

Solutions:
- Don't even go into the cafeteria with your homemade lunch.
- Eat outside if the weather permits.
- Find a spot with friends and share some conversation with your lunch.

Display your lunch to your friends. This sounds silly, but there is good reinforcement value to "showing off" a nutritious and unique variety of foods. After all, everyone knows that fast-food restaurants sell the same thing over and over, day in and day out. Your coworkers could tell you in their sleep what is on a McDonald's Big Mac because it is the same as a Big Mac in any city or suburb in the United States. But when you bring an avocado and turkey sandwich on seven-grain bread with a side dish of mango salsa and low-fat, blue corn chips, they will be curious. They may have never seen such a combination.

Another devilish solution to the cafeteria enticements is not to take any extra money to work or school. If you can't buy anything, these "fat-food" places can tempt you all they want, but you won't be able to substitute anything for your homemade lunch.

Advertising

Ads bombard us with mouthwatering, unhealthy choices. The food pictured in the ads on TV and in magazines is perfectly made, perfectly colored, perfectly stacked, and giant-sized to perfection. Real food you make is no match for that perfection. Think about it—sometimes real food is not pretty. It cannot compare to the food we see in ads.

Solutions:
- The more you follow the Family Day Planner and increase the time spent on family activity, the less time you will have for watching TV, a prime source for these ads.
- Stop leaving magazines around the house that have these food ads sticking out for the entire family to bump into.

Vacations

A huge mistake that families make while fighting obesity is that they treat vacation time completely different from regular home time—but a typical vacation of such time off puts on an average of seven pounds. Sure, you can and should relax some things during vacation time, but your commitment to your family's new activity and eating habits should remain firm. The weight you gain while on vacation may take as much as seven weeks to lose once you are back to reality.

Having the new attitudes toward food that we are outlining in this book, your enjoyment of eating and food will change. The fattening foods you once considered vacation-time treats will not be so appealing any longer. Keep this spirit going into your vacation.

Solutions:
- Change your thinking about vacation foods. You've had them countless times before. You know what they taste like; they haven't changed. They still have way too many calories and fat that you don't need. Just keep thinking about the weeks it will take to get that blob of fat off your thighs.
- Treat yourself on vacation in different ways. Get yourself a massage, a facial, or a makeover.
- Pack workout clothes.
- Keep up your family activity time.

A special note on the last point: Vacations are a good time to diversify your family activity by trying something new. In this way, vacations can be of great benefit to your Family Fit program. Actively encourage your family to try new things during these times. You may just bring home a new activity that will energize your fitness activity time and further motivate the family.

Traveling Away from Home

This dilemma is similar to vacations. Quite often, because you or your family are away from home, you try and comfort yourself by indulging in foods that you wouldn't eat while at home and practicing Family Fit.

Solutions:

- Plan ahead, know the enemy, and prepare yourself not to indulge in this way.
- Avoid going into places that will take you off your Family Fit Program.
- Don't carry "play" money around that will tempt you to buy fattening foods.
- At all costs keep up your activity level.
- Pack workout clothes.

Holidays

Holidays have been the biggest killer of weight control efforts. The indulgence of holidays started centuries ago primarily because it was only during holidays that certain foods were prepared and consumed. The gluttony of holidays came from the rationale that these special foods are around only once every year. This mind-set gave society permission to overindulge. In a way it is understandable that people would overdo it because these special foods wouldn't be available for long.

This tradition carried on, but in the last century our food storage capabilities have improved immensely, as has our transportation system, which has improved availability of foods. "Special" foods are rarely so special anymore in today's world. So the overeating excuse of "here today—gone tomorrow" just doesn't apply anymore.

> *Stop the common excuse: "I have to taste this because I haven't had it in so long!"*

Solution:
- You've had it before, and it tastes the same as it did back then. Once you allow yourself this excuse, a myriad of foods will pop up in your life that you haven't tasted or haven't had in so long. Stop!

Relatives

Your relatives will have lifestyles that they have determined are right for them. They will not necessarily know or practice Family Fit. You will encounter eating and activity habits at your relatives' homes that can trigger you back into obese behavior. This is because while at a relative's house you will be surrounded by all those influences and enticements that you cleaned up because of this program.

Solutions:
- Let a relative know in advance that you are following a new lifestyle program.
- While you are staying with a relative, take control of what you can to stay on the program.
- Plan an escape route; that is, make sure you can leave if the temptation is too strong to resist.

Stress/Emotional Eating

It is commonly known that stress causes overeating. Stress and emotional eating are very dangerous triggers because we tend to begin overeating before we realize what we are doing. Use stress and heightened emotional states as "red flags." When you are emotional or stressed, imagine a red flag in your mind and repeat to yourself, "This is a time when I am very vulnerable to go off my Family Fit Program." As was pointed out earlier in the book, remember that stress can be from negative sources and positive sources.

Solutions:

- Cope with stress in a new way. The best new way is to seek out help and support from another person. This person doesn't necessarily have to be a family member. Turning to others is the best overall coping mechanism for stress.
- If you are stressed, another excellent coping mechanism is to change the scenery. Get out of the environment you are in by literally moving to a different place. By forcing your mind to cope with a new set of surrounding environmental stimuli, your stress level lowers, and by physically moving your body, you discharge energy. Stress builds when the energy it creates in your body is not released.
- Do a fitness activity when you are stressed. This will add to your overall fitness effort and will have the same effect as changing the scenery.

Exercise

Yes, our old friend exercise can be a trigger for overeating. Exercise increases appetite; in particular, exercise makes the body crave carbohydrates to replenish those depleted by the workout. Because sweets are carbohydrates, many people who exercise crave sweets after a workout.

Complicating the picture is the fact that people who are just beginning an exercise program will fall into this carbohydrate craving more intensely than someone who has been active for years. Furthermore, many very intelligent people allow themselves an unhealthy food because they rationalize: "I've just worked it all off." The problem here is that people fool themselves into thinking they have spent more calories than that candy bar contains. They are always wrong, and they end up gaining weight after all that exercise.

Solutions:
- Be aware of your body's needs. Prepare for the cravings after a workout.
- Most of all, follow the Family Day Planner; it has placed the activity segments carefully to fend off after-activity overindulgence.

Gifts

You get an unhealthy gift and you feel compelled to consume it because, well, it was a gift.

Solution:
- Is it really a gift in the true definition of that word if it is unhealthy for you? Or is this well-meant gift just a Trojan horse in disguise? Take it back to the store where the giver bought it and buy something healthy. Better yet, politely and with great thanks give it back to the giver and explain to him that you and your family don't eat this type of food anymore.

The Fast-Paced Life

Rushing around or being overwhelmed with work demands or just the tremendous demands of modern family life can trigger unhealthy behavior. It is fast and convenient to stop at the fastest of the fast-food places to grab something to eat because there is just no time in the day.

Solution:
- Even at fast-food restaurants you can find a healthy choice if you read, think, and plan what you are going to buy. If you have the kids in tow, do not bend to the whines and wants of the children, who are more susceptible to the marketing lure of the fast-food restaurant!

THINGS TO REMEMBER:
- Avoid triggers that lead you back to bad habits.
- There is nothing wrong with avoiding situations—you are in control.
- Do not stop your Family Fit Program because you are away from home.
- Emotional eating is dangerous because it is an unconscious trigger—put a red flag up in your mind to remind yourself you're in dangerous territory.

CHAPTER NINE

A Short Course on Parenting

Any program that aims to involve and change the family has to address the issue of effective parenting. Whether it is a health-related program, such as Family Fit, a program to increase family communication, a program to increase academic success, or a program to establish better discipline in the family, all of these endeavors have to employ effective parent leadership and courage to change.

In reviewing many family programs of all types that try to establish change, it is astonishing how few of them take the time to explain how parents can accomplish these changes through better basic parenting skills. Most of these programs will detail their program with great enthusiasm and then stop and essentially say, "Now go ahead and start doing all those things." Okay...but many parents may respond to this with, "How do I bring together this disjointed family in the first place?" Here we will discuss the basic principles of effective parenting so that implementation of our family program is accomplished through the foundation of a more stable household.

This chapter can help supplement programs that address other concerns in your child's life. The principles here are not just for conducting a family fitness program.

Parents complain that they have little or no effect on influencing the choices of their children. Parents feel that what little effect they have dwindles as children grow up, culminating in teenagers who are totally independent creatures influenced only by peers and popular culture.

Parents may feel this way, but in reality several major studies that have come out in recent years have shown that parental influence *is* the most powerful determinant of a child's behavior. This makes parental influence stronger than peer pressure, media, music, and video games.

> *The first fundamental principle of effective parenting is to accept that you are the biggest influence in your child's life.*

In the recent past, parents have abdicated their influence over their children to these other influences. Parents have used these as excuses, and this allowed them to stop trying to influence their children.

> *Good parenting is leadership.*

Parenting leadership, like all leadership, comes at a price for the adults. Leadership is responsibility and work. Leadership is sacrifice and patience. Leadership is modeling and teaching.

Ben and Cecile do it right. They have three small children all under the age of eight. When they eat out and one of the children misbehaves at the restaurant, either Ben or Cecile will stop his or her meal and escort the misbehaving child out of the restaurant. They do this whether or not the meal is finished. Sure, the parent suffers because of the misdeeds of the child, but the loss of one meal out of a lifetime of meals is less important than the lesson of proper behavior and discipline in a public place. Actions such as this will pay big dividends in future years and will probably prevent the need for discipline in future situations.

Ben and Cecile demonstrate another important concept in parenting. They don't make a scene at the restaurant. They don't yell or slam their forks down or exhibit some other forceful adult behavior to emphasize parental displeasure. Their actions are controlled and firm, and they take action when they discipline the children. This highlights the fundamental parenting concept that:

Effective Parenting Is Businesslike

Parenting that involves adult hysteria is ineffective. When you lose control of your emotions as a parent, the only result is two people who are out of control. Sure, many generations of parents have yelled at their children, but we now know how powerless this is.

Think about it. What is the first reaction you have if your boss begins yelling at you, berating you, and demanding you change? For most people their first reaction is to tune out the boss's words. You just return to the same way you have been doing things.

No More Yelling!

If we could turn down the volume in families, there would be much more discipline and control in the households of America. Try it. Next time you want your child to do something you asked and he just hasn't done it, turn off the yelling. Stop what you are doing and approach your child face to face. Insist that he do what has been asked of him. If he does not get up right away and begin the task, stand in front of him with arms folded until he starts to move. Stand directly in front of the television or turn down the stereo until he moves to do the task. Then follow him as he does the requested task.

Why? First, the child's reaction (not performing the task when asked) shows you that he is not capable of handling that responsibility. This does not make him bad, delinquent, rebellious, or defiant. This makes him immature. If a child is immature and cannot do something, it is the proper role of the parent(s) to guide him step by step through the task. And don't do this with anger or frustration; just realize that this is a little child who needs to be taken by the hand and guided. Do this no matter what the age of the child—well into their teens if need be—because at any age, this is immature behavior. Parent this way and you will see the child's immature behavior change very quickly.

After reading all this, the first thought in many parents' minds will be: "Great! If I have to stop what I am doing and take little Susie by the hand until she does what she is told, I may as well do the job myself."

There are several responses to this thought. First, okay, doing it yourself is your choice. Second, this businesslike approach of firmness will take less time in the long run than starting the endless chain of screaming back and forth that can last all evening. Third, taking the child by the hand is parental *leadership*, and this makes the interaction between you and the child a teaching moment. Fourth, yelling will not change future behavior, thus making your life harder in the long run, but this new approach will change future behavior, which will make your life easier.

Parenting Means Sacrificing Conveniences

The idea that parents have to pay a price or become uncomfortable when parenting is a seldom-discussed aspect of the responsibility of parenting. Maybe it's a cultural phenomenon of present-day society, but parents always appear to be looking for the most convenient way to raise their children that doesn't disrupt their lives. But this Holy Grail of raising a child without changing your lifestyle just does not exist. No amount of nannies, baby-sitters, day schools, child psychologists, or whatever else can prevent you from changing your prechild lifestyle. Understanding this is so important for the success of the Family Fit Program.

Family Fit gives you a framework as a family to make family life organized and to create cooperation. Surrender your fantasy that family life will allow you to "do your own thing," and give in to making your family a support to your individual goals of health and fitness.

You may be thinking, "Okay, I can get my child to do what I want, but what about the other generations I want to get involved in the Family Fit Program?" The same principle of leadership applies here as well. Be insistent, don't argue or yell about involving them, and be businesslike.

Parenting Takes Courage

The scenarios presented so far all require parents to be courageous in their actions. It is hard to be in control and businesslike in the face of oppositional children. But once you see how successful the businesslike approach is, you will be reinforced to keep parenting in this style.

Being powerful is not negative. Don't be reluctant to accept your power as a parent. Remember the opening point of this chapter: *Parents are the biggest influence on the lives of their children.* This is an awfully powerful position to have in someone else's life. In parenting it is a very desired position as well. *Let's hope that parents are powerful.* Powerful parents can protect the child from life's hardships.

Examining the parental power that is gained by the parent's tremendous influence on a child brings us to another fundamental concept of parenting. Our children, until they are adults themselves, scrutinize us constantly for clues on what it is to be an adult.

This is very important to understand, especially in the context of the Family Fit Program that you are going to start with your family. The *only* task of childhood and adolescence is to learn how to be an adult. They have nothing else to concern themselves with but that single goal. Everything that a young person has to do developmentally falls under that one basic task.

Consider all the possibilities: Education's focus is preparation for adulthood. Sexuality, dating, courtship, and relationships are all about becoming an adult and choosing your life partner. Entertainment, style, music, and dress are all ways that the child and teen learn coping mechanisms for the pressures they will face later in life. Conflict, rebellion, anger, sadness, loss, and failure are all necessary experiences to help the young person cope with similar situations in their adult years. All of these are subcategories to the main task of learning how to become an adult.

Setting an Example

The real problem of growing up is that we parents don't give our children a handbook on how to handle all of these things. In fact, most of us don't do a great job of even talking about these experiences with our kids. If they have no handbook and we don't talk about it, then how do they learn how to become adults? They are left to do this only by observation. They watch us like hawks. They know every move we make. What are our reactions to things? What things make us angry, sad, or happy? When we change they are puzzled—why would an adult want to make that change? They desperately need to know so that it gives them a key on how to get where we are—adulthood.

Ask a teacher or anyone who works with large groups of youngsters if this is not true. If a teacher changes her hairstyle, the students in her class are on her like flies. "Why did you do that?" "Nobody wears their hair like that anymore; why change?" Change from glasses to contacts and you get the same reaction. Young people watch us closely. This is the only way they get what they need to know.

The effort that young people put forth to observe us emphasizes the influence and significance that parents have on children. If a youngster has a negative role model for a parent, she may scrutinize other adults in her world, but for the most part the youngster observes her parents.

This brings us all the way back to the beginning of this book when we discussed how the cycle of obesity is perpetuated. Now, considering how closely our children watch our actions, there is little surprise that they will copy our eating habits. After all, this is how adults eat.

Observing Our Attitudes
Another key element of effective parenting is attitude. With all this scrutiny, adults' attitudes affect young people very powerfully. Young people are not just observing an adult's body language, habits, behaviors, and language; they are taking in the adult's attitudes as well.

Recall the couple walking down the hallway smelling the bacon? What if a child was walking with them? That child would absorb the attitude of his mom savoring the aroma of the bacon as if it were a special treat. The child may not be able to pick up the thinking behind Mom's reaction ("I can't have it because it is not good for me"), but surely the child will pick up the emotion of that reaction. Will this translate into the child's mind that he or she wants bacon? There is a very good chance that this is exactly what will occur.

Even more important is the attitude with which you approach your family members. Is it positive and inviting even in the face of difficulty? Or are you harsh and negative? This is where your parental leadership really comes into play. It should be quite obvious that your attitude should be accepting, respectful, positive, calm, in control, and loving in all situations. Seems too fantastic to be able to do? Think about how the *businesslike* approach and the *no yelling* can lead you into a new attitude toward your family that will incorporate all those qualities. It is not that fanciful of a notion. You can make it happen.

Another tool that can aid you in creating an attitude that contains all those positive things is to watch your *expectations* of your children. One of the biggest causes of conflict between parents and their children is that parents' expectations of their children are way too high and unrealistic, and the children's capabilities are much lower. When the child fails or doesn't perform a task in the manner that the adult would have, the adult gets frustrated at the child, the adult shows the child her frustration, the child gets mad, and we are off to the races in family conflict.

It's not that children don't want to, or refuse to, comply with expectations. It is often that they physically or mentally can't. Children are unfinished products, and as such there are certain life tasks that are out of their reach. To expect them to do something that adults find natural is unfair.

Lower Expectations, Keep Standards High
Standards are different than expectations, and you should never lower the standards you set for your family. Standards are sets of ideal behaviors that we strive to attain. Standards are out there in the stratosphere, beckoning us to try to reach them. Expectations are realistic assessments of the abilities of a family member. Our children will fail because they are not finished products. That observation is a realistic expectation. We should always encourage them to keep on trying to achieve. That philosophy is a standard to keep pushing them toward.

Our children will fail because they are not finished products. Accepting that principle of parenting takes understanding and patience. It is our job as parents to be there when they fail, to pick them up, help them learn from the experience and try again. And our attitude through all of this should be "that's okay."

A good way to help our children when they fail is to model how we handle our own failures. Let them know how it feels to fail and what you do when you fail. This gives them one of those great big keys to unlocking the answers to life. It also lets them know that failure is a part of life.

Sharing is a good technique to help a parent model desired behaviors. If you share how you would approach a situation or how you would feel about a certain thing, then children get good parental guidance. As parents share their feelings, stories, likes, and dislikes, they provide the child with a road map to adulthood. Parents are often too inhibited to share their own stories.

This act of modeling is an important part of parenting. If you want your child to act in a certain way, then you have to model that behavior. To encourage your child to enjoy physical activity, you have to model that attitude. To be honest there will be times that the attitude of enjoyment on your part will have to be an act. That's okay; in fact, it's healthy for you and the child.

Consistency Is Key

We never say this in polite company, but there are several aspects of parenting that are an act. At times disciplining a child means that you have to act firm even though the behavior you are disciplining is comical. But you have to enforce the rules to be consistent, so you act like a parent, but later behind closed doors you laugh about what your child did. Don't feel guilty about this. The important point is that you are being consistent with your household rules, and consistency is the golden rule of parenting. Childhood can be a confusing and chaotic time of life and that intensifies once the child becomes a teen. Consistent parenting helps to calm all that chaos because kids learn that they can count on your response to life.

> *Parental consistency calms the confusion and chaos that can take place growing up.*

Along with parental consistency, helping children develop a sense of *mastery* in life is key to traveling smoothly through the growing years. Mastery develops when a child experiences a role or life task, is successful at completing this role or task, and continues to feel successful when this role or task comes into his life again.

Think of riding a bicycle. Now, think back to the day when you made your first smooth ride, no wobbling, just steady riding making confident turns. You established *mastery* over this task of riding a bicycle. Now, this mastery over a seemingly simple life task such as riding a bike develops in the young child the confidence to try to succeed at other life tasks. These tasks are tried, the child succeeds, and mastery builds and builds. To an adult, accomplishing such simple life tasks as riding a bike may not appear to be such a big deal. But adults forget that at the time they were challenged with this task, *it was a very big deal.*

Mastery is a developmental task that is very apropos here within the Family Fit Program. This program provides ample opportunity for young family members to gain mastery. The Family Fit Program, in fact, may be one of the *best* opportunities for young people to develop a sense of mastery. The Family Fit Program offers the young person many chances to participate in adult decisions and activities and to do so within the framework of things they will enjoy.

Look for ways that allow your child to develop this sense of mastery. Let them take the lead in family activities, tasks, and roles in the family. The pillars of Family Fit and the tools that fortify them offer many unparalleled opportunities to help your children develop this mastery.

Like mastery, another vital virtue that young people must learn to develop is *responsibility*. The development of responsibility is a lost art in today's families. More often than not, families are taking away opportunities for young people to learn responsibility. Young people are being sheltered from life's responsibilities at an unprecedented rate. This sheltering of young people is a leading cause of many of the problems we face in youth. Responsibility is learned by a process of give and take. It is important to give out responsibility to young people slowly. If they handle it, then gradually add more and more.

Don't Shelter Your Child from Responsibilities

It is important that they face them and maybe even fail at them. As they start to fail, that's when a parent steps in and helps them. Remember learning to ride that bike? You have to let them wobble a bit, but when you see they are starting to fall, you make every effort to grab the bike and prevent them from getting hurt.

Responsibility is learned in just this same way. Let your child wobble as she faces that teacher without her big science project. Don't step in and make an excuse for why she didn't complete it on time. Let her feel the anxiety of confronting the teacher with her failure. Facing this responsibility will help prepare her for future responsibilities.

Like the process of developing mastery, actively look for ways in which your children can handle a responsibility no matter how small. The Family Fit Program provides many opportunities to handle responsibility. Watch how they handle it and apply the golden rule of responsibility development:

> *Act like an adult, get treated like an adult. Act like a child, get treated like a child.*

Responsibility development boils down to this simple philosophy.

A final key parenting practice is assisted by this same golden rule. This is *setting rules and using consequences*. Many parents ask how to best set household rules and enforce consequences. This golden rule applies. If you have behaved like a little child, the consequence is given in response to that childlike behavior. If you act like an adult, then the consequence need not be given. The best way to give consequences goes back to that principle stated earlier: be *businesslike*. The parent should face the child and give consequences that fit the unacceptable behavior. Giving out consequences for behavior does not require a big confrontation. It can be very matter-of-fact.

Dealing with Consequences

This is not politically correct to say, but consequences should hurt. When you decide on a consequence, make sure it is something that the youth is going to feel. If you send the child to his room, make sure that the room is a punishment. But how many of our children's rooms are really a punishment when they are banished to spend time there? Most of the rooms have all kinds of neat, stimulating things to do. How do you get around this? Simple—pick another room for them to be banished to.

Sometimes you have to experiment with the consequence you are giving. Try something different. If it wasn't that effective, try something new the next time. Does that make the consequence a waste? No, you are still establishing that you are the parent and you will be giving consequences for unacceptable behavior. Your children will get the message.

Use yourself as a tool in giving consequences to your children. For example, say your daughter was abusive in her language all day long and then later that evening wants you to give her a ride to a friend's house. A great response is, "You expect me to go through the trouble of disrupting my evening to give you a ride when all day you treated me like a jerk? No, I will not take you to Karen's house." Giving this message is fair and will teach the child to think ahead.

Some parents feel hesitant to apply consequences for behavior. They think to do so will alienate their children from them. This is a guilt trap that parents should avoid. A parent's role is leadership, and when you lead, children will respect you all the more. Quite often your children are looking for the rules and boundaries that define behavior. Remember the facts presented at the beginning of this chapter. The only job of young people is to learn how to get to adulthood. When you spell out rules and consequences, you provide them with exactly what they are looking for. Inside they will appreciate, obey, and respect you for it.

Parenting is a hard and time-consuming job. The Family Fit Program is an excellent tool to make your parenting easier. Consider the principles discussed in this chapter and try to implement them in your home. They will work if you practice them with confidence.

THINGS TO REMEMBER:
- Parents are the biggest influence in a child's life.
- Good parenting is leadership.
- Effective parenting is businesslike.
- No more yelling.
- Being a parent means sacrificing your own conveniences.
- Effective parenting takes courage.
- Lower your expectations but keep standards high.
- Children are not finished products.
- Share your own stories.
- Develop mastery in young people.

CHAPTER TEN

Positive Side Effects

Throughout this book the positive side effects of this program have been pointed out. To highlight these positive side effects, this chapter collects and summarizes them.

Family Discipline

In Chapter Nine, discipline was highlighted. The Family Fit Program makes discipline much easier. As your family becomes more cohesive by sharing the common goal of fitness, you will find that the need to correct unacceptable behavior in young family members will lessen. By participating in Family Fit, your children will be around for you to control and observe more. Their tendency to act out will lessen. Similarly, because the children will be around more, you will be more involved and knowledgeable about their lives. You will be able to prevent unacceptable behavior before it starts.

Communication
A very positive side effect of the Family Fit Program will be an automatic increase in family communication. Family Fit instantly gives the family something to talk about around the house. You will find that this topic, health and fitness, is valued in all generations. Instead of being shut out of your child's life, you will be instantly included.

You will find that as you talk about health and fitness more freely, it will be easier to discuss other topics as well. Communicating as a family is a learned habit; once you open up the network to do this, you will find it generalizes to other areas. It is much easier to ask, "How was school today?" when you begin the conversation with "How was your lunch?" Checking in with your family members gives you an instant conversation starter.

Developing Better Coping Mechanisms
Family Fit develops coping mechanisms for life. Health and fitness are certainly valuable methods of dealing with life's pressures, but in Family Fit you are also learning to rely on others. Family Fit also teaches sharing. Young people learn through Family Fit that sharing is a key to success in any endeavor and a natural activity between two people.

Working Toward a Goal
The Family Fit Program also teaches every family member the value of working toward success. In Family Fit you planned, organized, and took active steps to achieve success. This progress toward success is a good learning tool for any family member.

Developing Confidence

As family members take on responsibilities, accomplish goals, and learn new things, they will develop that important sense of mastery over the world that was discussed in Chapter Nine. Along with mastery, confidence emerges as family members believe in themselves and believe that they can cope with life's tasks.

Creating a Diversion

The Family Fit Program becomes a diversion from life's stress for all family members. It takes time to think and plan in order to prevent mistakes and to be ready for sudden events. The thought that goes into the Family Fit Program keeps your mind from focusing on problems or stress. This is the type of diversion that therapists try to teach their patients—divert your mind onto something that is pleasurable.

Let's examine more closely how powerful a diversion a simple activity can become. Consider a family that has two children playing soccer. Simply attending the games requires a tremendous amount of activity that demands your full attention, thus taking your mind away from the stresses of everyday life.

Look at the following steps needed to help two children participate in a soccer game:

- Schedule the time to get to the game.
- Think about the approaching time to leave.
- Clean uniforms.
- Prepare a healthy pregame meal.
- Check the weather.

- Prepare the game bag.
- Prepare spectator's bag.
- Get directions to the game.
- Load car.
- Pick up Grandma and Grandpa.
- Travel to the game.
- Watch and cheer on team.
- Make sure players drink at halftime.
- Clean off kids after the game.
- Organize everything you took and prepare to go home.
- Eat after the game.
- Take Grandma and Grandpa home.
- Once home, help the kids shower and change clothes.
- Change your clothes and freshen up.

Breaking down a simple event such as attending a soccer game takes a lot of thought and planning. These events may seem mundane, but when we break them down we see the effort it takes for parents to make these events happen for their children. What a great job parents do with the everyday tasks of family life!

All of this effort takes you away from whatever pressure there is at the office. It's hard to think about what's going on at the office when you have nineteen things to think about and accomplish just to get your family to a soccer game. What a great coping mechanism. Approach these events with that spirit.

Your daily fitness activities in the Family Fit Program can provide just as much diversion. Each morning you will need to think about mobilizing yourself for the day. In addition, you will need to think ahead to what you are going to eat. Life becomes more active and diversified.

New Positive Atmosphere at Home
A new atmosphere is created in the home, one that emphasizes affirmation and cooperation. No more competitiveness among family members. No more sibling rivalries. Family time is quality time together.

Kids
Developmentally, the Family Fit Program fosters mastery, responsibility, discipline, motivation, communication, coping skills, family cohesion, consequences, rules, boundaries, delay of gratification, forward thinking, and maturity. For many of these developmental tasks, the Family Fit Program can be the best source for accomplishing these milestones. This is particularly true in these modern times when the pace and atmosphere of family life may not provide opportunities to experiment with these tasks.

Seniors
The discussion of developmental side effects should examine the other end of the developmental spectrum—senior family members. Pulling senior family members into this program has been emphasized from the beginning. Including seniors has tremendous physical and mental benefit for them. On the emotional side, this inclusion gives seniors a better sense of purpose in life. They become more attached to life. They will become happier, more cooperative, and more enjoyable to be around. This program solves many of the critical concerns of the geriatric years. Food and nutrition are the number one concerns for

seniors. A pillar of the program addresses this concern directly. Security is the second biggest concern for seniors. Senior family members will experience an increased sense of security because they are being pulled more firmly under the protective umbrella of the family. Seniors will truly feel a new lease on life when they actively participate in this program. Finally, geriatric research shows that the need for increased affiliation with their families is the third biggest concern for people as they enter their senior years. The Family Fit Program has built in fun, motivating, and stimulating avenues for very intimate affiliation among all generations of the family.

Preventing Larger Family Problems
Possibly the most noble positive side effect of this program is the preventive work it will do to keep family members of all generations both physically and mentally healthy. The physical health benefits have been emphasized earlier in the book. The emotional side effects are just as exciting.

People of all ages suffer emotional turmoil because of stress. The inherent coping mechanism for stress that the Family Fit Program provides has been highlighted. But without the focus on the Family Fit Program, family members turn to negative coping mechanisms—drugs, violence, domestic abuse, alcoholism—the list goes on and on. In young people, getting them involved in this program has tremendous preventive power. It's guaranteed that a youth focused on health and fitness will not smoke, do drugs, or become violent but will do better in school, will respect life and others more, will be more socially aware, will cooperate more, and will be a better friend.

We always focus in this society on the small percentage of people who are damaged, and this is often our litmus test of how a program is working rather than the great job it is doing in preventing damage. This program will be judged the same way. People will obviously lose weight and become more fit. But the intangible side effects may go unnoticed. Keep them in mind as you are enjoying your family more than ever in this program.

Health Benefits

Fitness has been shown to reduce the risk of heart attack, diabetes, cancer, stroke, and bone loss; it also reduces the number of minor illnesses suffered throughout the year such as colds, flu, and headaches. Fitness and a healthy lifestyle keep blood pressure and heart rate low, both of which have positive prevention effects.

Recent studies have also shown that fitness and exercise have very positive effects on mental illnesses, such as depression.

Fitness in seniors helps reduce the effects of aging.

Energy Level

With the improvement in eating habits, the increase in metabolism, and the improved mental alertness that Family Fit brings to the individual, the overall energy level of the individual will rise.

> **THINGS TO REMEMBER:**
> - You are crafting a new lifestyle through Family Fit; there will be many beneficial side effects.
> - Change is okay, as it exposes you to new reactions and experiences.

PART V
REAL GENERATIONS

CHAPTER ELEVEN

Success Stories

The families that have already applied the principles outlined in this book have had great success in improving their lives. The following are just clips out of their lives that highlight their victories in the Family Fit Program. Our true success stories make headlines!

Enter the Family Fit Contest and Win Big Prizes!
The Comptons—Mary, 39; Mario, 38; Grandma, 64; Grandpa, 65; Uncle Jim, 31; Aunt Sue, 31; Kate, 12; and Billy, 14—started the Family Fit Program together. They decided from the start to compare their progress at the end of six weeks, two three-week cycles. Each person put in $25, and they purchased a gift certificate at the best clothes store in town. At the end of the six weeks the person

who lost the most weight would win the $400 gift certificate. At the end of that six weeks every one of the Comptons had lost weight and was fitter and healthier, so no one was disappointed that Grandma had lost sixteen pounds and won the gift certificate. Of course, being a grandma, she turned around and used the gift certificate to buy each family member a new piece of workout clothing. Everyone won!

Houston Grandparents Are Amazed at How Often Children and Grandchildren Visit!

Houston seniors Ed and Dorothy Buck moved to a senior retirement village several years ago. Prior to moving, Ed and Dorothy were visited at least three times each week by their children and their grandchildren. These visits were necessary because Ed and Dorothy were still living in the family house, a sprawling ranch-style home that had been in the family for several generations. Ed and Dorothy found themselves unable to keep up with some of the basic household chores that the big house demanded. Jim, Ed and Dorothy's son, would fix whatever was needed, mow the lawn, trim trees, or do whatever project popped up. While Jim did these chores, Sara, Jim's wife, would cook some meals for the days ahead, clean the house, and do other chores that were becoming more and more impossible for Ed and Dorothy. The three grandchildren would play in the big yard or wander off into the forest preserve close to the house. These visits were pleasant, but with all the tasks to be done, the actual visiting time was extremely small. Family interaction time deteriorated to a quick, "Hi! How's everything? What do you need?" The visits became drudgery for everyone except the kids, who delighted in their outdoor adventures while visiting Grandma and Grandpa. The house was eventually sold, and with the proceeds Ed and Dorothy bought a condo in the senior development close to Jim and Sara's home.

At first, after moving into the senior village, Ed and Dorothy seldom saw Jim, Sara, and the kids. Ed and Dorothy were busy getting acquainted with their new neighbors or participating in one of the many activities offered to residents. After a while, Ed and Dorothy missed seeing their family and even became bitter that they didn't visit as much as they would have liked.

One day, at a business lunch, Jim discovered the Family Fit Program through a colleague from Chicago. Jim noticed how this colleague picked through the food that was served during lunch, and Jim began to ask questions. This fellow's family had been participating in Family Fit for months, and he bragged about the fitness benefits. While the man talked, Jim was also intrigued by how this man's family seemed to be having fun together doing this program. Jim asked if he could get a copy of the program, and the acquaintance e-mailed it to him the next week.

Jim brought the program home and Sara, always a fitness buff, immediately embraced it. Seeing how the program emphasized generational participation, Jim invited Ed and Dorothy to participate from the beginning.

Now, by participating in the Family Fit Program, Ed and Dorothy are with Jim, Sara, and the kids every day during the Family Fitness Activity segment of the program; quite often they stay to share a meal. What's more, these visits are now rich in interaction. No more is each family member isolated in his or her tasks. Ed and Dorothy have meaningful roles in the Family Fit program, and their health checkups have never been better. In fact, Ed, who had begun to use a cane when he moved into the senior village, doesn't remember where he last put that cane. His mobility and balance have improved tremendously.

Family Fights Exercise Guru and Wins!

The Ryersons are committed to their Family Fit Program. They have seen outstanding results in a very short time. They are much healthier; they talk and share together much more than they did before, and they feel as if they have a whole new life. The Ryersons are so enthusiastic that they cannot imagine leading their lives in any other way. One of the problems in implementing the program is that they travel a great deal, and they have faced several obstacles in their program while traveling. One of the biggest has been the attitude of hotels and the health clubs associated with the hotels they stay in.

Most health clubs have an age limit for using the health club facility. Hotels often set very rigid age limits for using the hotel's facilities. The Ryersons have two teenage sons who are strapping young men and excellent athletes. Both are well over six feet tall and have chiseled, muscular bodies. They look like full-grown men rather than the boys they are.

Both boys participate actively in triathlons and supplement their cross-training with weight circuit training. To keep up their level of participation, using a health club is essential. While at home, the Ryersons have made arrangements with a nearby health club to allow the boys to work out there. These arrangements were made when the boys were preteens. To get the health club to agree, it took Mom and Dad much negotiation, signing of waivers, and the guarantee that at least one parent is with the boys at all times while in the health club. This is no problem for the Ryersons because they are a Family Fit family, and they are participating in their fitness activity together anyway. These hurdles seemed ludicrous given the size and ability of these teenage boys, particularly in comparison to the majority of the patrons at this health club.

Unfortunately, when traveling, the Ryersons must redo these same negotiations, give the same evidence, and provide the same guarantees over and over again to each and every fitness "guru" at every hotel health club. When the Ryersons do obtain permission to use the facilities as a family, they are often the only people using the health club throughout their entire stay. The sad fact is that the Ryersons seldom get permission to use the health club. So the Ryersons are left with the alternative of trying to sneak into the facility, search around the area for a more enlightened facility, or do some patchwork weight training with whatever they can find.

This attitude *against* family participation in health clubs is a tragedy. These facilities should be the centers of family activity. Instead they separate families and do not encourage family fitness participation whatsoever. Consider how health clubs conduct children's swim lessons, one of the few times that a health club invites children into the club to use the facility. Most often during these lessons you will find the kids in the health club pool and the perimeter of the pool lined with parents in street clothes. *Wrong!* Get the parents into the pool with their children. Make this mandatory if they want their child to take the lessons. Although the Ryersons have to struggle for what they need, they successfully negotiate family participation most of the time.

Family Reins in Princess!

Jennie Sweeter grew up as an American princess. She was as cute as a button throughout her childhood. Because she was the only girl in a large family, her mother often treated her like a little Barbie doll. Most often Jennie could be found in frilly dresses and other feminine clothes. Jennie even participated in several Little Miss beauty pageants during her young life. With all brothers and all male cousins, she was considered a special gift to the Sweeter family.

Yet, with all of this attention and all of this maleness around her, Jennie was often a lonely child. With her brothers and cousins frolicking in boy's sports and games that she had no interest in, she often found herself playing alone. Indulged in childhood, she still wasn't happy.

Then as Jennie hit puberty, something frightful began to happen. For the first time, Jennie was plump. At the age of thirteen, she panicked. The one thing that always gave her self-esteem and accomplishment was now being taken away from her; the cute little Barbie doll body was starting to spread.

In the past, as the boys and their parents played together in vigorous activities, Jennie always felt these activities were beneath her. The rest of the family reinforced that attitude. They found it charming for this tiny princess to keep her distance in these family activities. From her toddler years onward she even had a response to her brothers' frequent invitations to participate in their physical activities. She simply said, "Why?" The rest of the family found the manner in which she said this adorable and even in this she was rewarded for staying along the sidelines of the family fun.

Now, with this crisis of puberty, Jennie saw how her brothers were all fit and lean, so she started to join in the physical activities of this energetic family. Soon, the crisis was abated. Her body became toned and shapely. Even more remarkably, she became happier and less lonely. By participating in the activity with the rest of the family, she felt a sense of belonging that she never had before. Instead of entering the tough teenage years with a great deal of unresolved childhood baggage, Jennie faced these years with a new happiness and energy that came through participating with her family in their fitness activities.

Sixteen-Year-Old Won't Eat Meat! Parents Shocked!

Cliff was a bright, energetic young man full of life and ready to take on the world at sixteen. One day at the dinner table, as a big beef roast was being served to the family, Cliff announced that he didn't want any. In fact, he added, he was giving up eating meat altogether. Cliff's meat-and-potatoes family was shocked, and their first reaction was to forbid Cliff from doing this because they believed it was surely unhealthy. "You need meat to live!" was Cliff's dad's refrain. Cliff was even punished at times for his refusal to eat the portions served to him. Gradually, Cliff's parents gave up the battle to force Cliff to eat meat. They rationalized that this fight had been going on for months, Cliff was not showing any signs of degeneration, they would rather not continue to make dinnertime such a stressful event, and surely this was some adolescent rebellious phase Cliff was going through. They thought they would ignore his behavior and it would go away.

Interestingly, after two years of Cliff's commitment to eating differently, Cliff's family found themselves being transformed from a household that ate beef every night for dinner to a family that ate it once every ten days. There was no grand discussion or epiphany that stimulated this change in their generations-old habit. It was Cliff's example and leadership that subtly translated this to his parents. At Dad's last check-up, his LDL cholesterol level had dropped 50 percent.

Persistence Gets Spouse Involved in an Affair!

When Tom was in school he was always busy studying, so he never exercised or played any sports or other extracurricular activities. His wife, Mary Ann, a businesswoman, claimed she didn't have the time or the interest for a fitness activity. Tom and Mary Ann were headed for disaster. Both were extremely busy young professionals just starting their careers. Tom was a new attorney working at a large law firm, and Mary Ann was a gifted financial analyst at an international accounting firm. Both worked unheard-of hours throughout the week and often on weekends. Their new marriage was rocky due to the lack of contact between them, the absence of relaxation, and all the stress they were under. They began to argue when they were together, and their romantic life totally fell apart.

They went to see a psychologist about their marital problems. To their surprise, the therapist diagnosed their problem not as a marital one, but as a lifestyle failure. The psychologist prescribed participation in a daily fitness activity and insisted the couple do the activity together. Mary Ann protested the loudest at this solution. She had no interest in working out, nor did she have the time. She didn't have the foggiest idea of what to do in a health club, let alone to perform at the level needed to make it worthwhile. Session after session revolved around trying to get Mary Ann to realize that the point of this prescription was not about performing at some "level" but about just taking the time to do an activity together. Furthermore, doing a fitness activity would be a great stress reliever for all the tension built up in her body. She continued to resist the solution; although some may have judged Tom as the quintessential nerd, he started going to the health club alone. At the sessions, Tom would explain he did very little actual exercise in the health club; just the change in atmosphere and getting out of his business suit and into workout clothes made it a relaxing experience. In these sessions, both Tom and the therapist would coax Mary Ann to try it, but she was steadfast in her refusal to enter a health club.

Finally, at a charity benefit they attended, Tom and Mary Ann met the director of the health club and his wife. They spent the entire evening with this energetic, lively couple and had a delightful time telling stories, laughing, and being entertained by the charming twosome. On the way home, Mary Ann remarked how much fun the other couple was and that she would love to see them more socially. As fate would have it, the club director called Mary Ann on the phone two days later to invite her to a ladies-only "spin party" at the club, hosted by his wife. Mary Ann eagerly agreed to go, even though she was a bit puzzled at the reminder to wear her workout clothes. But Mary Ann didn't hesitate; after all, she thought, this was a health club party. Maybe the workout clothes were like a costume theme.

Mary Ann arrived at the spin party and was shocked to encounter a dozen or more stationary bicycles lined up in rows. She was even more shocked to be ushered onto one of the bikes right up front facing the health director's wife, whose bike was turned around facing the rows of other bikes. With wild abandon the leader guided the group of beginners through a light yet vigorous spin-bike workout.

Even though it was a beginner's workout, Mary Ann was so unused to exercise that her body felt like a rubber band after the workout. She also felt as if a six-hundred-pound gorilla had been taken off her back. That's how much tension she felt was lifted right out of her body. Mary Ann was hooked. To this day she attends at least four spin workouts each week. Tom still flops around the health club doing his own thing, usually while Mary Ann is in her advanced spin boot-camp class. Their marriage is better than ever, and each is a more relaxed, energetic professional.

College Student Shocked by Roommate's Bizarre Behavior!

Jake couldn't wait to get to college. He had heard all the stories—beer drinking, parties, girls, pizza, food orgies, the works. When he checked into his dorm room, he saw someone had already moved in. There was an Oriental tea service spread out on a cart in the corner of the two-bed room, and a long planter took up the entire length of the windowsill. Popping up from the dark, chocolate-colored earth were rows of perfectly straight, bright green grass. A huge wicker basket overflowing with all kinds of fruits and vegetables hung from the ceiling. Okay, Jake thought, I have a biology major as a roommate.

As Jake began to unpack, a tall young man walked in and introduced himself as Ben. Jake, known for putting his foot in his mouth, inquired, "So, a little anxious to get started on that biology career, eh?" Ben explained that these things had nothing to do with his intended major—they were the things he liked to eat. The planter contained wheat grass that he took daily, and he preferred tea to any other beverage. He did not drink beer and had given up soda many years ago.

As Ben went on about his lifestyle, Jake was ready to quit school. This freak was dashing all the illusions he had about college. At that moment, there was a knock at the door, and a tall adult bounded into the room. It was Tommie Day, the legendary basketball coach and an icon at the college. He came in to personally welcome Ben to the college. As it turned out, Ben was the number one basketball prospect in the freshman class. Jake was frozen in awe of this legend right in his room on his first day at college. Jake dreamed that during his time at the school he might be able to catch a glimpse of this great man, but to have him in his room was the thrill of a lifetime.

As the year went on the two roommates made a comfortable enclave out of that room. Jake was in charge of tending to the planters filled with wheat grass, and Ben stocked the refrigerator with juices he got from the basketball trainer. Jake had great fun in his first year in college and learned a new healthy eating lifestyle from Ben.

Youngsters Find Hidden Passageway in Condo Building!

The Symthe family grew up in high-rise condos in a rust-belt inner city. Their neighborhood was in transition and was often unsafe. They did not have recreation facilities anywhere close to their building. Their condo unit was small; not even the living room had enough space to move around in. When the Symthes decided to start their Family Fit Program, they were baffled as to how they could choose a fitness activity that was doable given the confines of their living conditions.

This dilemma kept them from starting the program. They did follow the eating suggestions, but they were stumped on how to include a family fitness activity. Then one day the elevators in the building broke down for the first time in all the years that the Symthes lived in that building. Sissy, the Symthes's twelve-year-old obese daughter, walked up the stairway to their condo unit and burst through the door, huffing and puffing from her exertion.

Seeing Sissy, who was in need of exercise, so spent from this activity gave Mrs. Symthe a brainstorm. Walking the stairs daily would be the Symthes's first family fitness activity. This was creative and easily fit into the Symthes's time schedule. They could start with just a few flights of stairs and then build up to longer walks. They could increase the pace and even make games out of the activity. An added benefit was that they didn't have to travel anywhere. They could just walk right out their front door: The stairwell was two doors over. All this time, the solution to their fitness needs had been just two doors away, hidden like a secret.

British Family Loses Two Hundred Pounds and Doesn't Even Look for It!

The Thompson family moved to Chicago from London last year because of Mr. Thompson's job. Not familiar with the resources in their new American home, they were looking for something to do as a family to increase family time. Many of the recreation choices the Thompsons found were not ones that they enjoyed back in London. A new friend gave them a copy of the Family Fit Program, and they liked what they saw so much that they sent copies home to their relatives. They were motivated to share it with their relatives after reading about the need to change older generations. The Thompsons' relatives in England saw this as an opportunity to stay bonded with the Chicago Thompsons. Not only did both Mr. and Mrs. Thompson's parents go on the Family Fit Program, but aunts, uncles, and cousins did as well. Everyone communicated by e-mail. A total of twenty Thompson family members participated in the Family Fit Program. After three weeks of participation, these twenty people lost a total of two hundred pounds. Of course, being British, they measured their loss in kilos. The Family Fit Program offered this family a new, innovative way to connect, even across an ocean, which was fun, unique, and beneficial to their health.

New York Family Turns Great-Grandmother into a Monster!

The Garcia family wanted Great-Grandma Garcia to participate in their new Family Fit Program, but she kept protesting that she was much too old to do "anything silly like that." After weeks of prodding, Great-Grandma finally did join her family one Sunday.

The Garcias started this Sunday off with a homemade family breakfast of fresh-made tortillas, scrambled egg whites, fresh tomato salsa, mangos cut in half and served with a fresh lime wedge, and fresh-squeezed orange juice. Great-Grandma enjoyed this breakfast a great deal.

Next, the whole family went to church together. After they returned home, they changed clothes and went outside for a power walk around the neighborhood. They walked for forty minutes at a brisk pace. During the walk they sang songs, talked, laughed, and pointed out sights in the neighborhood they often neglected to see when passing by in a car or bus.

After they finished their walk, the Garcia family relaxed at home, read the Sunday papers, and visited with Great-Grandma. Great-Grandma instructed the young Garcias on how to make *paella* for Sunday brunch, and the youngsters showed Great-Grandma how to make this dish healthier. That afternoon they ate the *paella* for brunch, and afterward they drove Great-Grandma home.

Since that Sunday, Great-Grandma has not only participated with the family in their Family Fit Program but has also joined the local YMCA and her church's senior fitness programs. Now, Great-Grandma is exercising ten times a week. Great-Grandma considers her fitness activity her only form of social life. The Garcias created a monster in Great-Grandma, and her life has benefited greatly. She has gone from not being active at all to juggling the conflicting schedules of all her fitness programs.

Single Mom Pushes Baby on Lakeshore!

Penny is a single mom living in downtown Chicago. She has no extended family living anywhere close to her adopted hometown. Before she became pregnant, she was an avid runner. While pregnant, Penny read about the Family Fit Program. She promised herself that her child would be raised in a healthy household. Penny agreed with the ideas that Family Fit taught her about family activity and eating. Because of this strong belief, Penny did a wise thing. Even though her infant son, Trevor, isn't aware of what is going on around him, she started to bring him with her every day while she runs on the lakefront running path in Chicago. Trevor rides in a jogging stroller while Penny runs. When Penny works out at her health club, Trevor sits in his stroller right beside her with the opening placed so he can always see where his mommy is.

Penny feels that if she is going to start a lifestyle that includes her child in her fitness activity, there is no excuse why he cannot be with her from the beginning of his life. Penny feels that she is building a rhythm to her and Trevor's lives, and this early inclusion is a vital part of this rhythm.

CHAPTER TWELVE

Family Fitness Myths and Facts

Fitness suffers more from the myths about it than does possibly any other health-care concern. Here we will list common myths and present the facts that dispel them.

Myth: The Food Pyramid is for everyone.
Fact: For many people, six to seven servings of grains, breads, and cereals are too much. It can cause bloat, fat, and ill health. Notice this book did not promote following the Food Pyramid.

Myth: There is one perfect diet that will work for everyone.
Fact: Biochemistry varies so greatly from individual to individual that this is just not true. The Family Fit Program doesn't offer a rigid diet plan but an approach that can be tailored to the individual needs of families.

Myth: Stress does not make you fat.
Fact: The hormone released under stress—cortisol—leads to carbohydrate craving and overeating. By the way, *stressed* is *desserts* spelled backward!

Myth: All metabolisms are alike.
Fact: Everyone's metabolism is different because each human body is unique. Family members will not have metabolisms that are exactly the same. Even twins do not have identical metabolisms.

Myth: A balanced diet provides everything you need to stay healthy.
Fact: For reasonable health this may be close to the truth, but for optimal health this is not possible. You can eat a balanced diet and still not get all the nutrients your body craves. Trace minerals such as zinc, magnesium, and cobalt are good examples of such nutrients.

Myth: Sugar makes kids hyperactive.
Fact: A correlation between sugar and hyperactivity has never been shown. Hyperactivity, like eating disorders, is a multidetermined developmental disorder. It is believed that hyperactivity, now known as attention deficit hyperactive disorder or ADHD, is caused by the absence of brain biochemicals, which causes an inability to focus and concentrate.

Myth: Kids need meat for healthy growth.
Fact: Kids need protein, but meat is not the only source of protein. Many vegetables have large concentrations of protein. Soy products are very high in protein. Fish is also high in protein.

Myth: Celery is a negative-calorie food.
Fact: No food reduces calories. There are some foods that have no calories. Celery *is* a very low calorie food.

Myth: Brown eggs are better than white eggs.
Fact: Unless clearly labeled as low-cholesterol or low-fat eggs, which are very recent arrivals on the marketplace, there is no difference between these types of eggs. The color has no extra health benefits.

Myth: Vitamins and other supplements are food *replacements*.
Fact: Vitamins and supplements are intended to boost the health benefits of our foods; they are not to be used as food replacements. Supplements cannot and do not provide dietary fiber, which is essential to digestive tract function, and other essential building blocks that the body needs. Pills do not substitute for food.

Myth: Croissants eaten plain are a healthy breakfast.
Fact: Croissants contain twelve times the fat and 50 percent more calories than an English muffin or plain toast. Always read the nutritional labels on breads, as they are not all alike.

Myth: Chinese food leaves you hungry in an hour.
Fact: There is no scientific proof of this. Many Chinese dishes are heavily laden with rice and steamed vegetables and are low in protein, so you may feel hungry because you have a protein deficit by the time you digest that meal.

Myth: Eating late at night makes you fatter.
Fact: Families love to debate this issue, but the fact is that the time of day you eat does not have an effect on gaining weight. Weight gain still boils down to how many calories you eat in the course of the whole day. It is true that you burn fewer calories at night because your BMR slows when you are resting or sleeping.

Myth: Fresh fruits and vegetables are healthier for you than canned or frozen ones.
Fact: With modern freezing and canning procedures this is simply not true. In fact, frozen fruits and vegetables are typically picked at the peak of ripeness and then immediately canned or frozen, so these choices may have more consistent nutritional value than those you pick fresh at the grocer.

Myth: Fatty foods fill you up.
Fact: Fiber is more important in filling you up than fat. Fat does contain a higher percentage of calories than either carbohydrates or proteins, but the degree of fiber in all three categories of food varies.

Myth: You have to eat perfectly in order to lose weight.
Fact: There is no such thing as perfect eating. If perfect eating implies denial or sacrifice, then this is not true. You can have fun with food and lose weight.

Myth: If left alone without any outside influences, a child will eat only what he needs and will not overeat.
Fact: The tendency to overeat is instinctual. Children will eat motivated by instant gratification and not necessarily based on the physiological signal that they are full. Children are more governed by instant gratification than adults, so one could argue that they have a greater tendency to overeat.

Myth: Children do not have to worry about counting calories.
Fact: Children should watch calories just as much as adults should. The percentage of overweight children is skyrocketing. Children should be raised in an environment that teaches them to maintain a proper weight by watching what they eat.

Myth: Nuts are terrible foods that ruin diets.
Fact: Nuts are rich in unsaturated fats, not saturated fats. Eat small quantities because nuts are high in calories, and try to stick with the unsalted variety. Eating nuts can ruin diets because they are often eaten to excess, adding extra calories to the day's total.

Myth: If you eat a lot of salt, it automatically raises your blood pressure.
Fact: Although large quantities of salt are not good for you for a variety of reasons, high blood pressure is not one of them, says the latest medical research, unless you are salt sensitive.

Myth: Tea and coffee are the same for you healthwise.
Fact: Tea has less caffeine than coffee, and tea is a good antioxidant. Tea also reduces plaque in arteries. Tea does not promote bone loss. For all of these reasons, tea is a better health alternative than coffee.

Myth: Coffee needs to be eliminated from a healthy lifestyle.
Fact: The latest findings show that coffee in moderation is not bad for your health. The notion that coffee causes heart disease, stomach ulcers, and cancer has never been proven by research, and coffee is one of the most studied beverages.

Myth: Obese people do not burn calories as efficiently as thin people.
Fact: Studies show that the difference in calories burned by thin and obese individuals is very small and that any difference between the two is probably attributable to the extra weight an obese person carries around.

Myth: Strength training will stunt a child's growth.
Fact: Strength training will not slow or stunt a child's growth. It will help muscles grow strong as it is intended to do. The warning about strength training is about injury rather than slowing growth.

Myth: Artificial sweeteners cause cancer because of the phenylalanine they contain. The warning labels on diet drinks say so.
Fact: Phenylalanine is an essential amino acid that the body needs; it is also a component of the sweetener aspartame. Most people do not need to worry about this, but those who suffer from a metabolic disorder called PKU cannot process phenylalanine, and it will rise to toxic levels in the body. This is true for about one in fifteen thousand people.

Myth: If you drink a diet soda with a candy bar, the calories in the candy bar are cancelled out by the diet soda.
Fact: No drink or food can cancel out the calories in another food.

CHAPTER THIRTEEN

Outside Resources for the Family

In addition to all the facts and research compiled in the pages of this book, the following are sources of information you should know about. Many of these sources update information regularly. As your family continues to maintain their Family Fit lifestyle, continue to check for new information coming out on the positive fitness lifestyle.

American Academy of Pediatrics
141 Northwest Point Road
Elk Grove Village, IL 60007-1098
847-228-5005
www.aap.org

American Association for Leisure and Recreation (AALR)
Also houses the American Association for the Advancement of Health Education
1900 Association Drive
Reston, VA 22091
703-476-3490

American Council on Exercise
5820 Overlain Drive, Suite 102
San Diego, CA 92121-3787
800-825-3636

American Dietetic Association
216 West Jackson Boulevard
Chicago, IL 60606
800-366-1655
www.eatright.org

Children's Nutrition Research Center
www.bcm.tmc.edu/cnrc/

Consumer Reports on Health
P.O. Box 52148
Boulder, CO 80322
800-234-2188

Exer-safety Association
2044 Euclid Avenue
Cleveland, OH 44115
216-687-1718

Fat City
(Consumer diet fraud watchdog group)
www.healthwatch.org/dietfraud/
fatcity.html

**Fitness Motivation Institute
of America**
36 Harold Avenue
San Jose, CA 95117
408-246-9191

Food and Drug Administration
www.fda.gov

Food Guide Pyramid
www.nal.usda.gov:8001/py/pmap.htm

Gatorade Science Institute
www.gssiweb.com

Harvard Heart Letter
164 Longwood Avenue
Boston, MA 02115
800-829-9171
www.countway.harvard.rdu

iVillage Health Topics
(Variety of health/weight loss/
diet topics)
www.ivillage.com

Mayo Clinic's Virtual Cookbook
(Recipes for healthier meals and chat
site to share recipes)
www.mayo.ivi.com/mayo/recipe/
htm/maintoc.htm

Overeaters Anonymous (OA)
P.O. Box 44020
Rio Rancho, NM 87174-4020
www.overeatersanonymous.org

**President's Council on Physical
Fitness and Sports**
450 Fifth Street NW
Suite 7103
Washington, DC 20001
202-272-3421

Shape Up America!
www.shapeup.org

**USDA's Center for Nutrition Policy
and Promotion**
www.usda.gov/cnpp

U.S. Government Dietary Guidelines
www.health.gov/dietary guidelines

BIBLIOGRAPHY

American Academy of Pediatrics, Elk Grove Village, IL. www.aap.org.

American Dietetic Association (ADA), Chicago, IL. www.eatright.org.

American Psychiatric Association. *Diagnostic and Statistical Manual of Mental Disorders*, 4th ed., text revision (DSMIV-TR). Washington, D.C., 2000.

Food and Drug Administration, Washington, D.C. www.fda.gov.

National Center for Health Statistics (NCHS), Hyattsville, MD. www.cdc.gov.

Tamborlane, William V, ed. *The Yale Guide to Children's Nutrition.* New Haven: Yale University Press, 1997.

U.S. Department of Agriculture (USDA) and U.S. Department of Health and Human Services (HHS). *Dietary Guidelines for Americans.* Washington, D.C.: USDA, 2000.

U.S. Department of Health and Human Services. *The Surgeon General's Call to Action to Prevent and Decrease Overweight and Obesity.* Rockville, MD: U.S. Department of Health and Human Services, Public Health Service, Office of the Surgeon General, 2001.

U.S. Government Dietary Guidelines. Washington, D.C. www.health.gov/dietary.

USDA's Center for Nutrition Policy and Promotion. Washington, D.C. www.usda.gov/cnpp.

INDEX

A

activity pillar, *see also* Family Day Planner; fitness activity
    Family Day Planner form for, 158–159
    family goals, 67, 91, 144–149, 160–161
    generational goals, 67, 91, 144–149
    importance of other pillars to, 61–67
    individual goals, 67, 91, 144
    suggested activities, 148–157
adult leadership, *see also* parenting, effective
    for fitness activity, 144
    food protests and, 124–126
    importance of, 40–42, 47
    older generation and, 55
adults, obesity in, 16–17, 22
advertising, as bad habit trigger, 166–167
affirmations, 131–133
alcoholic beverages, 112–113
anorexia, *see* eating disorders
artificial sweeteners, 216
aspartame, 216
attention deficit hyperactivity disorder (ADHD), 212

B

babies
    attitude toward fat, 19
    developing tastes of, 20
bad habits, *see* habits, triggers for bad
balsamic vinegar, 102, 111
basal metabolic rate (BMR), 104–106
behavior, modeling of, 135–140
    effective parenting and, 178–179
    example of, 139–140
    failure and, 181–182
    self-motivation and, 136–138
blood pressure, 215
body language, *see* language
body mass index (BMI), 107–108
body weight set point, 33, 35
breads, 101, 110–111
breakfast
    in Day Planner schedule, 70, 76
    diet/nutrition tips for, 120–122
    habits regarding, 52
    nutritional balance and, 106
breast-feeding, 116–117
bulimia, *see* eating disorders
butter, 110–111

C

cafeterias, as bad habit trigger, 165–166
caffeine, 101, 215
calories
    calculating number of required, 104–107
    fat and, 99, 104
    myths and facts about, 214, 215, 216
    rate of burning, 31
candy, 110–111, 216

carbohydrates
  at breakfast, 120–121
  suggested scheduled for eating, 70, 71
celebrations, see social events/celebrations
celery, 212
cereal, 120–121
cheese, 100, 112–113
children, see also babies; parenting, effective
  body mass index (BMI) for, 107–108
  caloric needs of, 105
  eating disorders and, 34, 35
  family social situations and, 26–27
  fat and, 99
  fitness activity and, 145
  immaturity of, 176
  minor illnesses of, 125
  myths about calorie counting, 214
  myths about overeating, 214
  myths about strength training, 216
  numbers of overweight, 16, 22
  program's benefits for, 191
  program preparation and, 40–45, 59–60
  teaching to be adults, 178–179
Chinese food, 102, 213
cholesterol, 97, 98–99
cigarette smoking, change in attitude toward, 21–22, 65
cleanup, of home environment, 108–119
  drinking water, 115–117
  family planner food list for, 46
  as fortifier of diet and nutrition pillar, 67, 91
  removing/substituting foods, 43–45, 47–48, 110–113
  taking vitamin/mineral supplements, 117–119
coffee, 101, 215
communication, as program benefit, 188
confidence, as program benefit, 189
consequences, for children, 184–186
consistency, of parents, 182
coping mechanisms
  diversion as, 189–191
  improved, as program benefit, 188
  program as positive, 192–193
cream, 101, 110–111
croissants, 213
cycle of obesity
  effects on society, 15–17
  example of, 11–15
  family discipline/attitudes and, 18–20
  fitness activity levels and, 20
  genetics' role in, 31–33
  hand-me-down eating and, 17–18

D

day planner, see Family Day Planner
dehydration, 116, 127
desserts, 101, 110–111
  inappropriate use of, 19

diet and nutrition pillar, 129.
　　See also Family Day Planner
　adult responsibility for,
　　124–125
　breakfast tips, 120–122
　cleanup and, 67, 91, 108–119
　dinner tips, 123–124
　forward thinking, 67, 91,
　　119–120
　importance of other pillars to,
　　61–67
　lunch tips, 122–123
　new habits, 67, 91, 95–108
　snacks and, 126–128
diets, traditional
　Family Fit differs from, 106
　flaws of, 21, 30, 39
dinner
　diet/nutrition tips for,
　　123–124
　habits regarding, 52
dips, 112–113
discipline, see adult leadership;
　　parenting, effective
diversion, from stress, 189–191
drug abuse, contrasted to obesity,
　　16, 22

E

eating
　as basic human drive, 23, 25
　emotional, 24, 170
　handling protests about,
　　124–125
　importance of eating together,
　　51, 52–53
　importance of enjoying, 96
　late in day, 213
　myths and facts about habits,
　　211–216
　psychology of, 23–24, 35
　sociology of, 24–29, 35
　success stories of changes in,
　　202–203, 205–206
eating disorders, 34, 35
eggs, 121–122
　myths and facts about, 213
electrolytes, 116
emotional eating, 24, 170
energy level, improved, 193
exercise, see activity pillar;
　　fitness activity
exercise programs, weaknesses of
　　traditional, 68
expectations, of children,
　　180–181
extended family, see also older
　　family members
　as bad habit trigger, 169
　controlling influence of, 63–66
　handling those not on
　　program, 27–29
　preparing for program, 40–43

F

facts and myths, 211–216
　calories, 214, 215, 216
　celery, 212
　children, 214, 216
　eggs, 213
　fats, 214
　Food Pyramid, 211

fruits and vegetables, 214
meats, 212
metabolism, 212
nuts, 215
salt, 215
stress, 212
sugar, 212
vitamins, 213
family, *see* extended family; older family members
Family Day Planner, 67–68, 90
blank worksheet, 88–89
display of, 133
fitness activity and, 150–159
flexibility of, 72–73
structure explained, 68–77, 82–83
week one samples, 78–81
week two sample, 84–85
week three sample, 86–87
Family Planner forms
activity, 158–159
food list, 46
habits, 49
how to talk, 57
things/activities, 50
fast food, served in cafeterias, 165–166
fast-paced life, as bad habit trigger, 171–172
fats
calculating grams to consume, 99
cholesterol and, 97, 98–99
importance of, 96–97
myths and facts about, 214
reducing in diet, 100–103
types of, explained, 97–98

fitness activity, *see also* activity pillar; Family Day Planner
as bad habit trigger, 170–171
as diversion, 191
increasing intensity of, 82
midweek, 76, 77
on Saturday, 71
society's lack of, 20
stress and, 170
success stories of, 201–202, 203–205, 206–207
taking Monday off from, 75–76
varying on vacation, 168
water and, 116
food, *see also* eating; meals
examples of high fat, 44
healthy alternatives, 46, 111, 113
psychology of, 23–24, 35
social uses of, 24–29, 35
throwing out unwanted, 43–45, 47–48, 110–113
Food Pyramid, myths and facts about, 211
40-40-20 balance, 70, 96–99, 106–107
forward thinking attitude
benefits of, 58–59
as fortifier of diet and nutrition pillar, 67, 91
importance to nutrition, 119–120
fried foods, 102, 110–113
frozen foods, healthy, 123–124
fruits, 214

fun
    food preparation and, 114–115
    as program's guiding philosophy, 62, 96

G
gender, obesity and, 15, 22
generations, *see* extended family
genetics, role of, 31–33
gifts, as bad habit trigger, 171
goals, as program benefit, 188
grandparents, *see* older family members

H
habits, *see also* habits, new; habits, triggers for bad
    examining/changing of, 48–51
    myths and facts about, 211–216
habits, new, 95–108
    balancing carbohydrate, protein, fat intake, 96–99, 106–107
    calculating Body Mass Index, 107–108
    as fortifier of diet and nutrition pillar, 67, 91
    reducing fat intake, 100–103
    watching calorie intake, 104–107
habits, triggers for bad, 165
    advertising, 166–167
    cafeterias at work and school, 165–166
    exercise, 170–171
    fast-paced life, 171–172
    gifts, 171
    holidays, 168–169
    relatives, 169
    stress/emotional eating, 170
    travel, 168
    vacations, 167–168
hand-me-down eating, 17–18
HDL cholesterol, 97, 98
health, program's benefits to, 193
health clubs, attitude against families, 200–201
holidays, as bad habit trigger, 168–169. *See also* social events/celebrations
hot dogs, 100, 112–113
human drives, 23
hyperactivity, 212

K
kidney stones, 117
kitchen
    as home's center, 25–26
    replacing habit of sitting in, 48

L
language
    affirmations and, 131–133
    identifying harmful, 53–55

importance of using genuine, 141–142
messages about food and, 64
using helpful, 55–57
laughter, inappropriate, 53–54
leadership, *see* adult leadership; parenting, effective
lunch
    cafeteria food and, 165–166
    diet/nutrition tips for, 122–123
    habits regarding, 52
    midweek, 76–77
    nutritional balance and, 106
    on Saturday, 71

M

magazines, 51
mastery, developing in children, 182–183, 189
material rewards, 140–141
mayonnaise, 101, 112–113
meals
    common sayings about finishing, 14, 55
    preparation of, 51–53
meats
    myths and facts about, 212
    reducing fats in, 100, 110–111
mental attitudes
    forward thinking, 58–59, 67, 91, 119–120
    of parents, 179–180
metabolism, *see also* calories
    basal metabolic rate (BMR), 104–106

differences in, 29–30
myths and facts about, 212
milk, 100, 110–111
modeling of behavior, 135–140
    effective parenting and, 178–179
    example of, 139–140
    failure and, 181–182
    self-motivation and, 136–138
Monday-Monday excuse, 69
Mondays-Fridays, suggested schedule for, 75–77
monounsaturated fats, 97
motivation pillar, 142. *See also* Family Day Planner
    affirmations/surroundings and, 67, 91, 131–133
    importance of other pillars to, 61–67
    modeling behavior and, 135–140
    person-to-person motivation, 67, 91, 134–135, 141–142
    self-motivation, 67, 91, 136–138
    without material reward, 140–141
multimeal programs, 126–127
myths and facts, *see* facts and myths

N

negative reinforcement, avoiding, 134–135
nuts, myths and facts about, 215

O

obesity, *see also* cycle of obesity
    in adults, 16–17, 22
    in children, 16, 22
    current trends in, 17, 22
    in genders, 15, 22
    as social problem/contrasted to drug abuse, 16, 22
    treating as serious health concern, 64–65
older family members, *see also* extended family
    common sayings of, 55
    fitness activity and, 144–147
    gaining cooperation of, 64–65
    how to speak to, 54–55
    including in program preparation, 59–60
    program's benefits for, 191–192
    role of in program, 136–137
    success stories of, 198–199, 208–209
omega-3 fats, 97
omega-6 fats, 97
omelets, 121–122

P

pancakes, 121
pantry, cleaning out, 44
parenting, effective, 173–174
    attitude about, 179–180
    attitude about food, 19–24
    businesslike approach to, 175–177, 180, 185
    consequences for children, 184–186
    consistency and, 182
    expectations of children, 180–181
    improved discipline and, 187–188
    leadership and, 174–175
    mastery development in children, 182–183, 189
    power of, 177–178
    responsibilities of children, 183–184
    sacrifice of convenience and, 177
    uselessness of yelling, 175–177, 180
pasta, 100
peanut butter, 101, 110–111
person-to-person motivation, 67, 91, 134–135
    genuine language and, 141–142
phenylalanine, 216
physical activity, *see* activity pillar; fitness activity
physiology, differences in individuals', 29–31
pillars of Family Fit Program, *see* activity pillar; diet and nutrition pillar; motivation pillar
pizza, 102, 112–113
polyunsaturated fats, 97
popcorn, 103
potato chips, 112–113
potatoes, 101, 112–113
poultry, 100
pregnancy
    vitamin supplements and, 118
    water and, 116–117
    weight gain and, 19

preparation for program
   changing language, 53–57, 60
   cleaning house, 43–48, 60
   examining/changing habits, 48–51
   extended family and, 40–43
   importance of, 39–40
   including all ages in, 59–60
   preparing meals, 51–53
   thinking ahead, 58–59, 60
prepared foods, 110–111
preventive power of program, 192–193
proteins, importance of, 71
psychology of eating, 23–24, 35

R
race, obesity and, 16
refrigerator, cleaning out, 44
relatives, *see* extended family; older family members
resolve, about new lifestyle, 42–43
responsibility, developing in children, 183–184
restaurants, avoiding fat in, 102–103
rice, cooking, 100

S
sacrifices, parental, 177
salad dressings, 102, 103, 110–111
salads, in restaurants, 103
salt, myths and facts about, 215

saturated fats, 97–98
Saturdays
   beginning week on, 68–69
   suggested schedule for, 70–75
sauces, 102, 112–113
self-motivation, 67, 91, 136–138
set point, body weight, 33, 35
shortenings, 100
smoking, change in attitude toward, 21–22, 65
smoothies, 121
snack cakes, 112–113
snacks, 126–128
social events/celebrations
   as bad habit triggers, 168–169
   food's use at, 24
   incorporating into program, 73–74
   planning what to eat at, 27–29, 58–59
   suggestions for handling, 64–66
sociology of food, 24–29
   family gatherings and, 26–29
   food as coping mechanism, 24–25
   kitchen as gathering place, 25–26
sodas, 110–111, 216
sour cream, 112–113
special events, *see* social events/celebrations
speech, *see* language
standards, keeping high, 181
strength training, myths and facts about, 216
stress
   as bad habit trigger, 170
   coping with, 59, 170

Stress (*continued*)
   diversion from, 189–191
   myths and facts about, 212
success stories, 197–210
sugar, myths and facts about, 212
Sundays, suggested schedule for, 75
supplements, *see* vitamin and
   mineral supplements
syrups, 121

T
taco shells, 102
tastes, of children, 18, 19–20
tea, 215
teenagers
   caloric needs of, 105
   checking in with, 72–73
   eating disorders and, 34, 35
   immaturity of, 176
   role in program, 136–137
three pillars of Family Fit
      Program, importance of
      all, 61–67. *See also* activity
      pillar; diet and nutrition
      pillar; motivation pillar
trans-unsaturated facts, 98
travel, as bad habit trigger, 168
triggers, for bad habits, 165
   advertising, 166–167
   cafeterias at work and school,
      165–166
   exercise, 170–171
   fast-paced life, 171–172
   gifts, 171
   holidays, 168–169
   relatives, 169

   stress/emotional eating, 170
   travel, 168
   vacations, 167–168

U
unsaturated fats, 97–98

V
vacations, as bad habit trigger,
   167–168
vegetables, myths and facts
   about, 214
vitamin and mineral supplements
   avoiding excess, 118–119
   importance of, 117–118
   myths and facts about, 213
   pregnancy and, 118
vocabulary, *see* language

W
walking, 149
water
   as appetite suppressant, 117
   importance of drinking,
      115–117, 127
   kidney function and, 117
weekdays, suggested schedule
   for, 75–77
weekends, suggested schedule
   for, 70–75
weight loss programs
   difference of Family Fit, 106

flaws of common, 21, 30, 39
workouts, *see* activity pillar;
    fitness activity

Y
yelling, uselessness of, 175–177
yogurt, 102

ABOUT THE AUTHOR

Dr. John Mayer has been helping families with this positively centered approach for more than twenty years. A graduate of Northwestern University Medical School in Clinical Psychology, Dr. Mayer is a Diplomate/Fellow in both clinical psychology and sports psychology. This is the highest distinction one can achieve in these fields, and to have achieved it in two fields is rare. Dr. Mayer has built a national reputation for helping families. He consults across the country and is often called in on the "headline" cases involving youth. His newsletter, *Dr. Mayer's Memo*, is in its fifteenth year and is widely acclaimed for helping families and schools. This newsletter is distributed from coast to coast.

The American Food Service Industry has twice recognized him for his service to that organization in helping to serve the needs of youth. Dr. Mayer has been a pioneer in the weight loss field, having served as the psychological consultant to the first medically managed (OPTIFAST) fasting program in the Midwest. Dr. Mayer is nationally known for his work with addictions in families; consequently, for years he has treated patients for obesity and eating disorders as a form of addictive behavior. Through this work with eating disorders and obesity, families have successfully used the program and techniques in this book to live healthier, more fulfilling lives.

In addition to his professional life, Dr. Mayer and his own family are a testament to the success of this program. Dr. Mayer is an avid athlete. He is married and has two college-age children. His entire family is fit, healthy, and happy. They enjoy many activities together.